HIV and AIDS
A Social Network Approach

HIV and AIDS
A Social Network Approach

Compiled by Roger Gaitley and edited by Philip Seed

St. Martin's Press
New York

First published in the United States of America in 1989

Printed in Great Britain

ISBN 0-312-04045-8

Library of Congress Cataloging-in-Publication Data

HIV and AIDS

Includes bibliographical references.
1. AIDS (Disease)--Social aspects. 2. Social sciences
--Network analysis. I. Gaitley, Roger II. Seed,
Philip
RC607.A26H56   1989   362.1'9697'92   89-10932
ISBN 0-312-04045-8

CONTENTS

'Every moment we can choose our point of view, we can choose to see AIDS as a grim crisis for humanity or as an extraordinary opportunity, individually and collectively, to move forward. We can allow it to confirm our powerlessness, despair, hopelessness, isolation and terror of being all we can be, or we can use it as a springboard from which to make the boldest, most graceful leap towards living the life of our dreams and getting our world exactly right.'

Christopher Spence

Director, The London Lighthouse

Acknowledgements

Chapter 2 was researched and compiled by Martyn Hall who was, at the time, a social work student at Aberdeen University. He is now a qualified social worker. The remaining chapters were researched and compiled by Roger Gaitley.

Grateful thanks are extended to Martyn for his valuable contribution. Sincere thanks must go to the staff and clients of 'Maynard House', the members of the 'Bridge Group' and 'Kirsty', 'Mike' and 'Beth' Rankin. It is not possible to identify those who have helped by so freely giving of their time and life stories. It is abundantly obvious, however, that this book could not have been written without them. They, along with all of those living with HIV and AIDS have shown that it is possible to live satisfying and full lives despite the virus and that they along with friends, partners and families are in the vanguard, meeting with success the many challenges posed to the individual and society by this disease.

Social Network Analysis

The case material in this series is based on social network analysis. During the past decade social workers and others in the helping professions have stressed the importance of understanding social networks. For example, it is important to recognise the importance of informal care as well as formal services.

Social network analysis is a new method of systematically measuring social networks. Part of this method consists in asking clients to keep diaries for a monitored period, usually a fortnight. Some months later the exercise is repeated. The diaries are focused on finding out the people, places and activities that are important to clients in daily living. Services are then evaluated in this context. Other 'information components', as they are called, include details of the client's social setting, the client's views and the views of the client's main support person at home (e.g. parent in the case of a child, son or daughter, perhaps, in the case of an elderly person) and assessments of the client's features of performance in interests.

Social network analysis is useful in research, for management and for monitoring services, as well as for individual practitioners. Its research applications are expressed in *Applied Social Network Analysis* (Costello, 1987). Its use for practitioners is described in a forthcoming book *Introducing Network Analysis in Social Work* (Jessica Kingsley, 1989). Dr Philip Seed is the author of both books.

Editor's foreword

The preparation of this book has entailed close collaboration between Roger Gaitley and myself. The bulk of the work has been undertaken by Roger - he is an authority on social work with HIV and AIDS. My contribution, apart from editing, has been to offer the theoretical framework of social network analysis which Roger at once saw to be highly relevant to his topic. Network analysis brings out the potential strengths in a client's situation, emphasises client views and an understanding of his or her lifestyle. It emphasises the potential for hope based on health.

Into this framework, Roger brings a breadth of understanding which is unusual in the literature to date on this subject. Whether it is the intricate social implications of the infections or the benefits of a wholefood diet or safer sex or drug use, Roger writes authentically. He also knows about social work and the networks of available support in the health and social services and from voluntary groups.

The implications of HIV and AIDS bring us face to face with the WHO definition of health as a state of physical, mental, social and spiritual wellbeing. The resources bearing on all of these aspects of human functioning need to be mobilised not just by health and social service workers, but by managers, policy makers, and the community as a whole. Prejudice based on ignorance has no place. Whatever our personal views on this emotive topic, this book provides the means to become much better informed. At the same time it must be stated that this book does not attempt to deal with the ethical dimensions of sexual relationships, although there is scope for discussion of these issues as they arise both with regard to interpersonal relationships and the wider role of state and other societal institutions to intervene. In common with other books in this series, each chapter ends with a section on points for discussion.

Chapter 1

Introduction

A small but very telling cartoon appears in a book *Living with AIDS* - a guide to survival written by 'Frontliners' (a group of people diagnosed as having AIDS). The cartoon depicts two children, one of whom is saying to the other 'Hey! Let's play insurance agents and people with AIDS!' The other replies 'Oh goody! I'll fetch the bargepoles.'

Encapsulated within this cartoon is the reality that people living with HIV (the human immuno deficiency virus which can cause AIDS in an unpredictable number of people with the virus - see *Appendix A*) know only too well. The reality for them is living daily not only with the medical uncertainties posed by this virus but also with the stigma, discrimination, and ostracism caused by popular reaction to the virus.

Any examination of the social and epidemiological history of HIV and AIDS since 1981 will show how the virus has brought together a veritable pot-pourri of intense social taboos such as 'deviance' (primarily sexual and drug using), a handicapping and so far incurable disease in mainly young people, dying and death. It is not, therefore, surprising that the virus has had such a profound effect not only on the lives and social networks of people with, or at risk of, HIV infection but also on their partners, families, friends and social carers, both formal and informal.

Fear of HIV and AIDS

The bargepoles of the cartoon are undoubtedly the bargepoles of fear, which have a double-sided dimension - namely, the fears of people who have HIV, and the fears of the rest of society about people with HIV and their own perceived risks of infection.

These fears can potentially undermine the very fabric of social networks and relationships; for the person living with HIV and AIDS, the dimensions of fear may be such that they end up leading isolated, unhappy and depressing lives. Aspects of these fears most commonly associated with HIV infection have been:

1. For people with HIV

- acute fear of AIDS (sometimes known as AFRAIDS).
- development of psychosomatic symptoms which mirror those associated with AIDS, i.e., night sweats, tiredness, loss of body weight, skin disorders.
- fear of loss of physical and mental control.
- fear of a painful death.

- fear of the unknown (the future, after death, etc.).
- learned fear due to internalised oppression (often associated with sexual lifestyles).
- fear of other people's reactions (particularly rejection) which may lead to a deliberate choice to isolate oneself sexually and socially from other people.
- fear leading to conscious or unconscious denial of AIDS.

2. For people without HIV

- acute fear of AIDS (developing symptoms as already described).
- fear of infection due to perceived risk sexual behaviour (often referred to as associated with the 'guilty worried well').
- homophobia - a fear of gay people.
- fear of situations inappropriately associated with putting oneself at risk of contracting HIV, i.e., visits to the dentist, giving blood or receiving blood transfusions, social contact with people who have, or are thought to have HIV.
- fear leading to denial of the possibility of HIV. 'Despite what I do it will not happen to me.'

3. For carers of people with HIV and AIDS

- fear of being swamped emotionally and practically.
- fear of being out of control and de-skilled.
- fear of drug users and gay people.
- feelings of unease about issues associated with drug use, sexuality, dying and death.
- reluctance to care because of one's own prejudices or those of one's own family and friends

Any appreciation of these fears, therefore, requires people living with HIV and AIDS, carers, friends, lovers, family and society in general to investigate the dark alleyways of their minds in which these fears may have taken hold. Without this there can be no doubt that unfulfilled lives will be led, social networks will be potentially distorted and unconditional compassionate care will not be given to people with HIV and AIDS.

There have been many tragic examples of the way fear of HIV and AIDS has intruded on and upset social and community care plans for people with HIV or AIDS. For example, the failure of the Milestone Trust's plans to open a hospice for people with AIDS due to the prejudice about, and ignorance of HIV which characterised the opposition of the villagers of Torphichen. The London Lighthouse residential support and care centre had to contend with the initial anxieties of the residents of North Kensington who did not wish to be on the same sewage and water supply as a centre caring for people with AIDS. In prisons, inmates with HIV are invariably isolated. In hospitals, patients with HIV and AIDS are commonly barrier nursed. These, and many other examples, stand as a stark and daily reminder that help and support for people with HIV and

AIDS has to confront and, indeed, can be tinged by, experience of intense social and emotional alienation - an alienation which has rocked the delicate balance between the issues of public health and personal rights.

Living with HIV and AIDS

To understand the effect on social networks of a diagnosis of HIV, it is important to stand back for a moment and consider what it must be like to face the diagnosis with its prospect of a life of potential uncertainty with a virus for which there is currently no known cure or vaccine, and for which such conventional palliative treatment as exists may have unpleasant and very toxic side effects.

It is an understatement to describe the experience of people who have discovered that they have HIV as traumatic and devastating. A gay man writing in a bulletin of the Sussex AIDS helpline describes it very well:

'When I saw the doctor he told me that I was in fact antibody positive. I felt the hairs stand on end, I was so deeply shocked. He explained the condition and talked about the future, but I didn't take anything in ... My initial reaction was one of complete terror. I was convinced that I would never have sex or a relationship ever again and, even worse, I thought that I was going to die. I felt totally immobilised and was unable to think about anything else. I turned to drink and felt isolated from all my friends, believing that none of them could understand my feelings ...'

With the support of understanding friends, parents, and 'Body Positive' (a support group for people with HIV) he was able to regain a sense of security, start going to discos for gay people and eventually feel able to find a new lover and partner. Personal respect was regained and a new sense of openness and sharing was achieved which helped his family to become a closer unit, although he was still experiencing some rejection from his father who did not find it at all easy to accept his son's antibody status and (by implication) his gay lifestyle.

People who discover they have HIV, in seeking acceptance and understanding may incautiously wish to disclose their status. This can precipitate adverse reactions because of the aforementioned fears and the associated stigma. It is natural to feel an intense need to tell friends, family, and colleagues at work, but these disclosures must be tempered by the following considerations:

- what are the advantages and disadvantages of such a disclosure?
- is the disclosure being made in order to seek love and support?
- why is it important for this particular person to know?
- how will this person handle the disclosure and the confidentiality required?
- how will disclosure effect social, physical and material wellbeing should the infection progress and symptoms of chronic HIV infection and AIDS develop?

Overall, it will be an anxious and very confusing time and it is important that the formal and informal carers are available, do not over-react but remain calm, are accepting and empathic in their care and seek to reduce personal and environmental stress as much as possible.

If this is achieved, the person with HIV and AIDS may well find that they are able to establish new networks and close friendships and, above all, live a positive and healthy lifestyle.

To achieve this lifestyle, however, personal and practical adjustments may have to be made. All the good will in the world will count for little if there is not an environment with adequate financial and residential resources within which a person with HIV or AIDS can live as independent and stress-free a life as possible and, if necessary, be appropriately cared for.

Networks

The basic premise that underpins all that is written in this book needs to be stated.

All care (informal and formal) for people living with HIV and AIDS or who may be at risk of infection (by virtue of their risk behaviour - not their implied membership of so-called 'risk groups') must be delivered in the context of as detailed an understanding as possible of all the factors that are important to that person's daily living. By taking account of people, activities, and environments, a total view will be arrived at of where a person obtains their key supports. This view must take into account all social, legal, health, and interpersonal networks, and where they complement, overlap, or even stand in contradistinction one to another. This viewpoint should also stand alongside an awareness of the progression (if any) of the HIV infection in that person's life. By bringing these views and understandings together a flexible augmentative social care planning programme should be achieved. This will retain the central focus on the needs and wishes of the person with HIV and AIDS. Without this approach, formal and informal care runs the risk of being not only demonstrably counterproductive but also intrusive to the point of further marginalising a person who, by social ostracisation, may already be found to be at the margins of society. Furthermore, by acknowledging that HIV has the potential capacity seriously to weaken social patterns, it is possible to discourage those patterns that can lead to further risk of infection while promoting the development of new patterns of safer and healthier living. This is particularly pertinent when considering the advocacy and implementation of safer sex and safer drug using lifestyles (see *Appendices B* and *C*).

An analysis of individual, or even organisational needs related to stages of HIV infection will tend to be clinically and disease determined. Therefore, any appreciation of need based on the environmental and social contexts becomes much more important. Such an approach has its roots well bedded in social work tradition.

Central to casework is the notion of the person-in-his-situation as a threefold configuration consisting of the person, the situation, and the interaction between them.[1]

The terms 'internal pressure' and 'external pressure' are often used to describe forces within the individual and forces within the environment as they impinge upon, and interact with, each other.

Hence, for any understanding of the needs of the person with HIV or AIDS or any self-help, statutory or voluntary agency that aims to help them, an understanding is required of the factors, influences, networks and psychological frameworks, of all the key people in the gestalt. Social network analysis is the key to this understanding, through a detailed study of all the coherent patterns that may be evident. Because there is increasing evidence that groups or networks may be as effective as individual counselling (if not more so) in engendering positive attitudes to living well and constructively with HIV and AIDS, it is of considerable importance to identify these groups and networks. Once identified, they can be placed firmly within the 'situation in life' of the person living with HIV and AIDS and their importance evaluated. The following chapters will, therefore, describe and explore these concepts.

In *Chapter 2* an agency and its work are described that starts from the experience of making contact at street level with 'rent' boys who may, by their sexual activities, become at risk of HIV infection. Boys are very vulnerable because of the interaction between poverty, the sexual exploitation they have experienced and their social and family networks.

Chapter 3 considers direct work being done with drug users at a city based agency, 'Maynard House.' Some of these users are HIV positive, are partners of people with HIV, or have, by their activities, put themselves at risk of contracting HIV. All have social, health, legal, and formal care networks that are crucial to whether they continue to live risk-free lives. An analysis of their networks shows the important aspects of daily living and focusses on the treatment plans for the individual as they see them and as their counsellors see them, and highlights any dilemmas. The chapter concludes by considering briefly the position of gay people in relation to HIV.

Chapter 4 focusses on the situation and the needs of infants with HIV and their carers. A case study describes the home life of one such baby who was fostered and then formally adopted by her foster parents. The networks of the adoptive family will be considered and, in particular, the family and health networks and support systems that are available for the child and family both on an individual and group level. The thorny issues around confidentiality and who needs to know about the child's antibody status are also examined.

Chapter 5 concentrates on a study of a group (The 'Bridge Group') set up to provide support for relatives of a family member who has HIV. Such groups, e.g. 'Friends', 'Positive-Partners' 'Terrence-Higgins Trust Family Support Network' recognise that, common to caring for people with HIV, must come a recognition of the raw emotions, stresses, and practical problems, common to the families and partners of people with HIV and AIDS which undoubtedly affect functioning and networking.

Chapter 6 focusses on the potential for social workers and other carers as HIV health promoters. This is a potential that is often denied because of bureaucratic role demarcation, feelings of ignorance and of being de-skilled. Often there is a painful denial of the need for the carers to start with themselves and examine how healthy and risk-free are their own lifestyles. There will be an examination of some of the aspects of living positively which come within the framework of holistic health and which can be seen to complement as well as challenge conventional medical therapies for HIV.

Given the uncertainties of HIV, *Chapter 7* looks briefly at how the principles and theories outlined in the book can be taken forward in the light of future developments in the care and treatment of HIV and AIDS and the potentially changing epidemiological progression of HIV infection.

Finally, whilst it is recognised that a detailed description of HIV and AIDS can be found in many other publications, it is necessary for the reader to have brief appendices outlining the key medical information needed including a glossary of terminology used and a summary of what is understood by safer sex and safer drug use. A brief bibliography of suggestions for further reading is included.

As is now the pattern with *Case Studies for Practice*, all the persons who have been interviewed and the agencies described have given their permission for the material that has been used. The personal information and networks drawn are authentic and only their names and the details of the agencies and support groups have been altered to protect confidentiality. The material that has been used has been based, in the main, on daily diaries which were kept over two periods of one week in the latter months of 1988 and January 1989.

This book is intended to be of use not only to social work students on CQSW and CSS courses but all those workers in voluntary and statutory agencies engaged in caring for people living with HIV and AIDS. Ultimately the book is dedicated to those children and adults with HIV and AIDS who, by their courage and example, have shown that in the face of misinformation, stigma and apparent hopelessness, it is possible to live well and positively. As Frontliners have again so succinctly put it: 'Even with AIDS all hope is not lost - there are more grounds for optimism than you might expect.'[2]

Reference

1. Hollis, F. *Social Casework - A Psycho-Social Therapy.* New York: Random House, 1964
2. Frontliners, *Living with AIDS - a guide to survival by people with AIDS,* 1987

Chapter 2

Making Street Contacts

'It doesn't do any good if you give people a message they don't listen to.'

- Dr Merv Silverman,
Public Health Director, San Francisco

This chapter describes the work undertaken by a social work student, Martyn Hall, to set up a health education project in central London with a voluntary, charitable organization which deals specifically with all aspects of Acquired Immune Deficiency Syndrom (AIDS) and Human Immuno-deficiency Virus (HIV) infection. The aim of the project was to promote and disseminate a risk-reduction message to young people on the streets in a city centre, particularly those involved in high-risk activities, *viz* unsafe (unprotected) sex and/or unsafe drug use (sharing 'works'). Specifically targeted were injecting drug users and prostitutes - both male ('rent boys') and female ('working women').

The account that follows is by Martyn Hall and was written early in 1988.

The agency in which I was working is a voluntary organization with a remit to 'inform, advise and help on AIDS'. The agency is young, having been formed in 1982/3. Initially a self-help organisation for gay men and those concerned with HTLV III (as the virus was then known) it has now become an internationally recognised support, advice and information agency. It runs a number of services for particular groups as well as a general provision for all sections of society. The work of the agency can be summarised under three headings: advice and counselling; support groups; information.

Advice and counselling

The agency operates a daily AIDS helpline which is known nationally and handles calls on all aspects of AIDS and HIV. There is a priority line for people with AIDS (PWA's)* and those diagnosed antibody positive (of which all London hospitals and sexually transmitted diseases-genito urinary medicine (STD/GUM clinics) have the number. 'PWA's is a self defining term by people with AIDS. Also, a 'Vistel' service operates for people with aural disabilities. Crisis intervention is available for short-term help for individuals with AIDS or HIV infection and if required, face-to-face counselling can be offered.

---

*The term PWA is tending to be less used. The term has been seen as rather impersonal and denies the ability to live a positive lifestyle irrespective of the disease - Ed.

Legal referrals can be dealt with, and practical advice and assistance given on housing and welfare issues. Drug referrals - both from agencies and self-referrals - are handled by the Drugs Education Group (DEG). The DEG provides information, support and counselling for users, as well as training other agencies on AIDS issues.

Support groups

Self-support groups are part of the agency's core policy and there are now such groups for PWA's (that is, people diagnosed as having AIDS or ARC - AIDS Related Complex) specific to people who are HIV antibody positive; drug users (past, maintained or active); women; lovers; families.

'Buddying'

Lying somewhere between counselling and support is the 'Buddying' service, which uses experienced, trained volunteers to visit PWA's (and if necessary their families, friends and lovers) on a regular basis. They will do, or help with, practical tasks such as housework which PWA's may find increasingly difficult, as well as make hospital visits and be available to talk about subjects a PWA may find distressing - such as illness and death. The role of the buddy is intended to complement and supplement the statutory services.

Information

The agency tries to provide a comprehensive and up-to-the-minute information service on all aspects of AIDS and HIV. Much of this is dealt with by the Health Education Group (backed up and informed by the Medical Group) through such projects as the 'Roadshow', a mobile health education/safer sex campaign originally based in a disco for gay men. Also, the agency produces a number of leaflets and booklets which are widely available, runs conferences, workshops and training and is able to provide speakers for many engagements. A number of advice and policy groups cover issues such as drugs, legal, religious, health, medical and welfare benefit problems and the question of how they might affect people with AIDS and HIV.

The agency, although it now has a full-time staff team, is still largely run by a large pool of volunteers. Some are highly qualified in their field; many offer simply commitment and enthusiasm. By maintaining this largely volunteer structure the agency keeps in touch with its principal ethos - self-empowerment and the rejection of passive compliance (both to the virus and to the statutory service provision which would consign people to the role of helpless 'victim').

Historically, the agency has directed its efforts towards gay men; more recently it has also devoted its attention to injecting drug users. The Roadrunners project was proposed to work with young people on the streets, in keeping with this concern to work effectively with marginalised groups. Such groups are alienated and therefore less receptive and more distrustful of any information, advice and/or initiatives from 'the establishment'. The project also recognised the unique vulnerability of such marginalised and alienated people who are involved in what can be termed 'high-risk activities'.

The Roadrunners project

When I arrived, the project was still only a proposal and its aims, objectives, rationale and implementation were mapped out in the following in-house document.

'Roadrunners'

AIMS: To make contact with young people on the streets, including male and female sex industry workers (prostitutes)

OBJECTIVES:

To inform and educate about the risks of HIV and AIDS

To develop a referral network for possible counselling

RATIONALE: Young people on the streets often inject and support their habit with prostitution. They are therefore at increased risk of HIV infection. It is highly unlikely that these people are being reached by the statutory services, and other organisations like CLASH and STREETWIZE are probably not large enough to make sufficient impact.

IMPLEMENTATION:

1. Formation of Roadrunners group using trained volunteers with street credibility if possible!

2. Contact building and liaison with other groups plus further training if necessary.

3. Printing of cards for safer sex and safer injecting.

4. On the road.

5. Evaluation - numbers of referrals - accceptance levels

BUDGET: 6 months - volunteers' travel costs £2,500 - printing of cards £2,500 (TOTAL £5,000).

It was from this embryonic stage that I had to set up and implement the project. My starting point was to arrange a preliminary meeting to get other people involved and to start some discussion to bring out ideas and suggestions. Information about the Roadrunners project was circulated to all staff and volunteers within the agency and also specific invitations were sent to a couple of relevant organisations with which the agency had close contacts. These included agencies concerned with action on street health, advice and counselling service for youth, and a health improvement team.

The outcome of this preliminary meeting was a great deal of enthusiasm and a number of ideas and recommendations which I could then work with. However, having drawn up the minutes of the meeting I felt that there was going to be a tendency to 'run before we could walk' and that, in fact, a great deal of preparatory work ought to be done to make us fully aware of all the potential problems so that we did not fall flat on our faces.

The proper beginning for a health education project - bearing in mind the words of Dr Silverman - was to look at where our targetted groups 'were at' in regards to AIDS and general health awareness. Everybody has now heard of AIDS and even if they know little or nothing about it, they have some notions or conceptions (or misconceptions) and generally hold some views and ideas about health and disease.

Lay theories about AIDS

Working at the Faculty of Education and Community Studies at Bristol Polytechnic, Aggleton and Homans have studied people's notions of health and illness, particularly in relation to AIDS and HIV, and have identified four types of lay theories about AIDS[1,2].

(i) endogenous theories

(ii) exogenous theories

(iii) personal responsibility theories

(iv) retributionist theories

Endogenous theories suggest that AIDS is caused by something within the individual, only requiring a set of circumstances to 'trigger' the illness. A 1986 study[2] showed that 44% of respondants believed that homosexuality *per se* caused AIDS. The significance of such beliefs is that a person's perception of whether or not they are at risk may be determined by whether or not they see themselves as being gay. (Indeed, some men may at times be involved in homosexual behaviour but not regard themselves as being homosexual.)

Exogenous theories see AIDS as caused by something external to the individual. This is a long-held view of illness causation that sees disease spreading like a mist of 'miasma' through the air. More specific to AIDS is the belief that HIV is highly contagious. The consequence of these exogenous views is a desire on the part of the holders to avoid certain persons and environments which they presume will increase the likelihood of their own infection.

Personal responsibility theories locate the cause of AIDS within irresponsible behaviour. The tendency here is to differentiate between what the media (and the Princess Royal) have termed 'innocent victims', suggesting that others, presumably, are 'guilty'. In this latter category are included gay and bisexual men, the sexually promiscuous, prostitutes and injecting drug users. Through their behaviour it is almost 'reasonable' that they should have contracted HIV infection. There are, of course, the 'innocent victims': haemophiliacs, blood and blood product transfusion recipients, and the partners and children of either injecting drug users or the promiscuous.

Aggleton and Homans draw an interesting distinction between these views, which are usually applied to others, and the beliefs people hold about themselves where illness, including AIDS, is largely dependent upon luck. There may be some point in trying

Models of intervention

There are two models of intervention that it is possible to use, which may be described as either 'shower' (i.e. top-down), or 'bidet' (i.e. bottom-up).[8] The shower model assumes a uniform community with only passive involvement and involves handing down information from above. Traditionally this model has been used for AIDS education and awareness, particularly by the government. This model will have some effect on the community, but by assuming uniformity (presumably in order to reach the largest number) marginalised groups are not reached and are further alienated by the assumption that they do not have specific needs. The bidet model, in contrast, involves a discrete community comprising both overlapping and separate groups interacting together leading to some intervention. In the case of this study, the community comprised former drug users and prostitutes (some individuals may be both) together with other women and men in the Roadrunners group for the purpose of initiating a health education project.

Using the bidet model we took our risk-reduction message back to contacts in the targetted groups to get feedback on how it should be phrased and presented to be 'user friendly' (to borrow a term from the computer world), and then back in the Roadrunners group work with this information.

The other aspect of presentation was how to produce material that took account of the fact that not everyone is literate (looking at current provision the assumption must be that only those who can read are at risk, or that those who can't do not matter!). Also, some people from ethnic minority backgrounds may not have a working knowledge of English (material has been translated - Hebrew, Arabic, Cantonese, Bengali, Urdu, Punjabi, Gujerati, Hindi, Turkish - but either does not take account of, or is hindered by, the necessity of making the information culturally acceptable, e.g., Muslim, Jewish and Chinese attitudes to sex in general and homosexuality in particular).

The result was to produce a short series of stickers using cartoon format, with as little written information as possible, portraying a 'Roadrunner' character who would be a drug using, non-gender specific/hermaphrodite prostitute. Various adventures or scenarios would be depicted and the message simple - safer sexual and drug using practices. As I left the placement the first graphic was to be produced the following week.

Newsletter

Continuing liaison was firmly established with our group of external agencies by the production of the first *Roadrunners Newsletter* to keep them in touch with us and with each other and to inform and update them on AIDS/HIV issues relevant to their work.

COVENANT HOUSE: an article on the work of Covenant House, New York City's largest shelter for runaway children, is featured in the January 1988 edition of *Psychology Today*.

Covenant House runs an outreach programme working with drug users, rent boys and women prostitutes on the streets. There is a concern that these adolescents will become part of a 'third wave' of the AIDS 'epidemic'. Risk-related behaviour puts them directly in the path of the virus - there is an 'epidemic of exposure'. However, adolescent exposure to the virus may not be readily obvious since any resulting conditions may not appear for a number of years when they are young adults.

AIDS AWARENESS: the same publication also quotes a University of California San Francisco (UCSF) study on AIDS awareness amongst adolescents. Only 60% knew that condoms may help prevent transmission of the virus; nearly 25% thought AIDS is curable in its early stages. Misinformation was highest amongst blacks and Hispanics.

NEEDLE EXCHANGE: the widely publicised figure of 1 in 61 babies being born with HIV antibodies in New York may not be replicated in the UK as a result of use of needle/syringe exchanges. The babies in New York are the children of drug injecting mothers.

Merseyside, with a high incidence of injecting drug use, has so far had no babies born antibody positive. Merseyside DDU believes that this is a result of their policy of exchanging old 'works' for new, clean sets, backed up by information on safer sex and the distribution of free condoms. Doctors working for Mersey RHA are also prepared to prescribe maintenance scripts, recognising that not all users wish to come off drugs.

A government survey shows the incidence of sharing works is declining. However, only 5% of injecting drug users are regular clients at exchanges.

YOUTH SERVICE RESPONSE TO AIDS: the National Youth Bureau has produced a curriculum pack for youth workers, managers and policy makers. Information in the pack includes:

- all age groups claim increased knowledge about AIDS, but there is no sign of appreciable behavioural change (BBC/Gallup Study)
- many young people are confused by the recent mass of AIDS/HIV information, largely because they lack basic knowledge of sexual and bodily functions
- information alone is not enough, discussion needs to take place
- injecting drug use appears to be increasing in Glasgow, Edinburgh and Merseyside and evidence suggests most users have shared 'works' at least once
- information does not take into account beliefs and prejudices people hold about health

The pack contains case studies of initiatives in Shrewsbury, Leicester, West Lancashire, Ellesmere Port and Alternative Youthwork amongst drug users on the Wirral (based on primary prevention, risk reduction and links with needle exchange schemes).

An AIDS resources list is also included.

SAFER SEX: the experience of San Francisco suggests that safer sex works. HIV infection has almost halted amongst the city's gay men. The 'safe sex' campaign appears to have been very successful in less than 4 years.

ROADRUNNERS: the administration and co-ordination of the Roadrunners project will be handed on to a full-time volunteer at the Trust at the beginning of February, 1988. Once it has been finalised who that individual will be, we will let you know so that liaison on the progress of the project will be continued.

FEEDBACK: has this newsletter been useful? How useful is the breakdown of the figures? Are we wasting our time? Any comments on the information included in the newsletter would be useful to us so that future updates are kept relevant. Perhaps there are areas or topics not included that you would find any news on useful? Please let us know.

The Roadrunners project was a particularly difficult initiative to work on. I knew little of how to set up a project and at first was unaware of the numbers of issues involved. Unfortunately, my major error was in assuming right at the very start that the original project proposal had been assessed as a workable idea. In hindsight I could have taken the proposal back to the Health Education Officer and discussed with her how she had arrived at the content of the proposal. This would have established the flexibility of the proposal and the degree of my autonomy as project co-ordinator. As it was, the problems and unworkability of the project were pointed out to me by outside agencies and at times I found myself defending an idea I had not properly looked at and discussed. Had I initially established that the proposals were not binding but simply suggestions as to how the project could be carried out and that I had the amount of autonomy and flexibility that it turned out I had, the early preparatory work would have been smoother and we would not have suffered the loss of credibility that we did. However, through time, patience, negotiation and communication I did manage to get all the agencies together and working in the same direction - a glaring gap, though, was not involving the needle exchanges which were used by at least 5% of injecting drug users. Recognising this, they were to be asked to participate. Generally, though, I was able to do a lot of work in setting up the project.

The most important parts of a health education project are to identify the message to be put across, who it is to be aimed at, and what are their special needs and situation. The work I did on the Roadrunners project covered these areas comprehensively. With my study of lay theories of health, I constantly referred back to links we had with the targetted groups in relation to the eventual format of the material. At the end of my three months we had a project that was workable, flexible, and agreeable to the agency, the Roadrunners group and the network of external agencies.

I had also been able to establish a group of volunteers that were committed to, and involved with, the project. I believe I was able to recognise and implement the main points of working with volunteers.[9]

- role clarification (both perceived and expected)
- communication
- understanding (of role, motivation and tasks)
- management (recruitment, selection and support)
- monitoring

It was to members of this volunteer group that I was able to hand over, with due preparation, the running of the project.

Perhaps the acid test of my efficacy is to look at what service was aimed at drug users and prostitutes on the streets before Roadrunners, and what there was three months later - a health education campaign, thoroughly thought through, and just about to be launched, and a specific AIDS/HIV liaison forum for the different agencies involved in working with these groups. I hope this will just be the beginning.

Postcript

One year later, in February 1989, Martyn Hall returned to the project to look at how the work had progressed, whether Roadrunners was a useful, viable project, and to see what problems and/or developments had occurred in twelve months. His report follows:

> What I saw and heard disappointed me, largely because of the time factor. The project has not progressed a great deal further. This, it seems, was not for the want of trying by those involved but because of problems within the project. Yet Roadrunners still exists as a project within the agency and its aims and objectives are still supported. Its development, though, has been slow and problematic.

This appears to be largely the result of a significant lack of support, from both within and outside the agency. Roadrunners is a project within the Health Education section of the agency and, therefore, the first base of professional support is the Health Education Officer. The departure of the HEO, (a short-term appointment) and then a period of vacancy meant that support has not been available. Equally, despite a commitment to running the project from a volunteer basis, there was difficulty in maintaining the established volunteer group (mainly it appears to do with individual circumstances) and this obviously created difficulties - particularly when the services of the cartoonist were lost.

The external agencies too showed varying degrees of commitment. A decided effort was put into maintaining the Roadrunners newsletter, but a lack of feedback led to the usefulness of this in terms of time and effort being questioned. Roadrunners still liaises with relevent agencies, some, such as Streetwise Youth Project have continued to express interest in, and support for, Roadrunners, whilst others, such as CLASH, have dropped their connections. Following the identification of agencies which ought, but hitherto had not, been included in Roadrunners liaison the project has not established useful and constructive links with other agencies.

Contact with local councils has been allowed to lapse since the production of early drafts of the cartoons made it appear increasingly likely that they would not be passed as acceptable by the councils but that, if the message were toned down to accommodate them, they would not be effective with the target groups.

The current stage of the project is that final drafts of three cartoons (one each aimed at male prostitutes, female prostitutes, and injecting drug users) have now gone for approval by the agency's viewing committee.

The issue of language and limiting written information has proved a problem and all three cartoons contain significant information written in English. The project is looking at the production of material with little or no writing for the future. The production of the cartoons has taken too long since we committed ourselves to circulating drafts to agencies to put to their client groups for comment on their effectiveness and acceptability. This proved to be very time consuming, and the lack of feedback already noted compounded the problem. It goes without saying that losing the services of the cartoonist held progess up considerably.

The material is now all but ready and locations to be targetted have been identified. A method of carrying out continual distribution of the stickers has been worked out.

Many of the original ideas of the project have been maintained but have proved, in effect, problematic. Roadrunners has also spent time and effort looking at new initiatives (e.g. development of 'smack-packs'* - papers that drug users could use for wrapping drugs in but which would have safer drug use information on - and also the possibility of a telephone answering service women prostitutes could use for safer sex information, and indeed encourage their clients to reinforce information about the necessity of using condoms). With all this in mind the local Health Authority have invited Roadrunners to re-apply for continued funding based on an evaluation of work to date.

Points for discussion

1. What are the advantages and disadvantages of using a student placement to start and develop a Health Education project?

2. Was the student's sense of disappointment in the postscript a year later justified?

3. Discuss the different lay theories of AIDS.

4. Discuss the complexities of working with other agencies in a project of this kind.

5. Health Education is only one part of the function of the Roadrunners' host agency. Is a multipurpose voluntary agency the best host for a Health Education project? Under what other auspices might it have been sponsored?

6. Discuss the merits of a cartoon approach bearing in mind the difficulties of communication in a multi-cultural environment.

References

1. Homans, H. Aggleton, P. et al. (1989), *Scientific and Social Issues*, Churchill Livingstone.
2. Aggleton, P. and Homans, H. (1987), *Educating About AIDS: a discussion document for Health Education Officers, Community Physicians, Health Advisors and others with a responsibility for effective education about AIDS'*, Bristol: NHS Training Authority pp 20-22.
3. Vass, A., quoted in Aggleton, Homans and Warwick, *op. cit.*
4. Zald, M. N., 'Sociology and Community Organisation Practice,' In Zald, (ed.), (1967) *Organising for Community Welfare*, Chicago: Quadrangle Books, p.55.
5. Smith, G., (1970), *Social Work and the Sociology of Organisations*, London: Routledge and Kegan Paul, p.109.
6. Ibid. p.58.
7. Rothman, J., (1974), *Planning and Organisation for Social Change: Action Principles from Social Science Research*. New York and London: Columbia University Press, p.126.
8. Wiseman, Tina. *Marginalised Groups and AIDS Education*.
9. Richards, K., (1977), *Training Volunteer Organisers*, London: National Institute for Social Work, pp 46-49.

---

*Smack - a colloquial slang word for Heroin - Ed.

Chapter 3

People living with HIV

The experience of living with HIV or the threat of HIV infection can, and often does, have a profound impact on a person's social network systems. These systems will invariably involve interaction with the family (nuclear and extended) and will certainly include friendship networks (sexual and non sexual), health networks, and, in many cases, involve contact with social care and/or legal agencies.

This chapter explores the experiences of four people in contact with 'Maynard House' (a social care agency for drug users, their families, and friends) and will conclude with a general discussion of the impact of HIV on the lives and networking of men and women who have sex with partners of the same sex.

Maynard House

Maynard House is a city centre drugs project which operates on a psycho-social model; that is to say, that both psychological and social factors are taken into account when working with individuals. The project operates on therapeutic community principles.

From its inception in 1983 Maynard House has always aimed at operating a structured counselling service for drug users as opposed to the predominantly crisis orientated approaches being adopted by most of the surrounding community based agencies. The project receives many direct referrals from prison and social services departments and has established very effective close working relationships with General Practitioners, community psychiatrists, local hospitals and health centres. Maynard House's working philosophy has led to the deliberate identification of the high levels of illness and offending among drug users and, as such, the service (mindful of the impact on the individual of 'labelling') has focussed on the labels which have a major impact on the lives of drug users, in particular such labels as 'patient', 'offender', 'addict', 'chaotic'. To this list can be added the stigma of being seen as high HIV risk.

The staffing of Maynard House comprises:

- project co-ordinator
- senior project worker
- four project workers
- secretarial and voluntary support workers

The increasing spread of HIV amongst drug users together with a realisation that it is risk behaviour and not membership of a 'risk group' that is the important consideration has undoubtedly had a major impact on the work of Maynard House since 1985. The attraction of government AIDS money has enabled the project to widen its *modus operandi*. The full range of work currently being undertaken by Maynard House can be described as follows:

1. Advice consultancy and training.

2. Sessional counselling around dependency and health issues (particularly HIV).

3. Offenders, prison consultancy and advice and a direct service to prisons, courts, and social services.

4. A day rehabilitation programme. (Initially this was a drug free programme but now people are accepted in the latter stage of a detoxification programme).

5. Sessional groupwork with particular HIV groups and family support groups.

The project takes referrals from a thirty mile radius of the city in which it is centrally based. A good network of bus and train services enables the clients to reach the project with relative ease. Maynard House has also initiated some outreach work into areas of the city suburbs where HIV infection amongst drug users is known to be prevalent and where continued needle sharing and associated HIV risk behaviour is thought to take place.

Maynard House offers an expert witness service to local courts and has begun to operate an offenders induction programme for people on a deferred court sentence. Such a programme may last up to 12 weeks. Independent assessment reports on drug users may also be provided by the project on request.

Maynard House uses the following model for referral:

1. Discussion with referrer about the client's, presenting problem. (Any work formerly done with the client will be identified).

2. An initial meeting with client and referrer.

3. A formal contract drawn up between Maynard House and client to which client, project worker and referrer are signaturies.

4. Regular reviews by all parties to the contract are also arranged.

In order to ensure that the aims of the project are adhered to and evaluated, and that the project workers function well given the stress of involvement in drug and HIV problems, at least six hours a week are devoted to staff support, case discussions, daily worker support meetings, individual supervision, and in-service training. The measure of personal and group support offered to the researcher during his visits to the project is evidence of a philosophy well inculcated in the everyday life of Maynard House.

Maynard House is therefore a very pivotal part of HIV work in its locality. (See *Figure 1.*)

Ryan

Ryan, a young man of 26, comes across as someone trying to take good care of himself and make a favourable impression. He dresses well and likes to keep fit by playing five-a-side football and attending a local gym for weight training. Neither activity is represented in his diary (see *Figure 2*) as during the week he completed his diary the gym was closed for repairs, and the football team had no match. Ryan's overall presentation is, however, far from 'macho' and his gravelly voice is indicative of years of heavy smoking.

Ryan has been diagnosed HIV positive for two years, the diagnosis being made shortly after that of his fiancée Dianne who had been tested positive at the same time as their son James. The drug using history of Ryan and Dianne, their residence in a run-down fairly impoverished area of the city well known for its drug using sub-culture and high level of HIV sero-prevalence had been indicators that had led to the testing of Dianne, James, and then Ryan for antibodies to HIV. Ryan has remained asymptomatic since diagnosis but Dianne has developed lymphadenopathy (see *Appendix A*), weight loss, and has at times been quite unwell. Despite the risk of repeated HIV sexually transmitted infection Ryan and Dianne will not contemplate safer sex and the use of condoms for sexual intercourse. James was born HIV positive but is now testing as HIV negative, having, it appears, thrown off his mother's antibodies to the virus. (The situation of chidren similar to James is explored in *Chapter 4*.)

Ryan and Dianne have been living together for seven years and were recently rehoused to a three bedroom council house on the edge of a run-down suburban estate about five miles from Maynard House. James does not live with his parents, but with Ryan's mother. James is currently subject to statutory supervision and care under child care legislation. As can be seen from Ryan's diary, much activity has been spent in decorating their flat and creating an environment conducive to the 'Authority's agreeing to allow them to care for James.' Ryan sees his optimum environment as one in which he does not offend, does not misuse drugs and has a clean and tidy home. Both he and Dianne are very motivated to convince staff at Maynard House, doctors, social workers and their family that they are doing well and will eventually be able to care for James.

Ryan has been using drugs since a teenager when he tried cannabis. By the age of twenty he was injecting heroin regularly as well as dipipanone (Diconal). Although the latter is meant to be taken orally, Ryan and his friends would crush up these tablets and dissolve them in water before injecting. Occasionally Palfium would be used and latterly Temgesics. ('Crap - I didn't really like them'). At the height of his drug use with Dianne, Ryan would require he reckoned £250 - £300 per day to finance their combined drug habit. Ryan freely admits that the social experience of 'shooting up' with friends was very important and as valid as the effects of the drugs themselves. Despite the fact that the syringes they used were usually not cleaned properly, the drugs mixed with impure water, and the level of purity of the street heroin available invariably very poor, Ryan, Dianne and the friends with whom they injected rarely gave any thought to the associated risks, specifically hepatitis, gangrene, overdosing and certainly not 'AIDS'

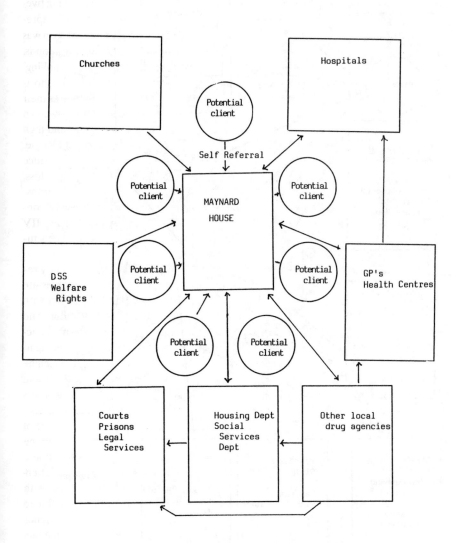

Fig. 1 - Maynard House Locality Network

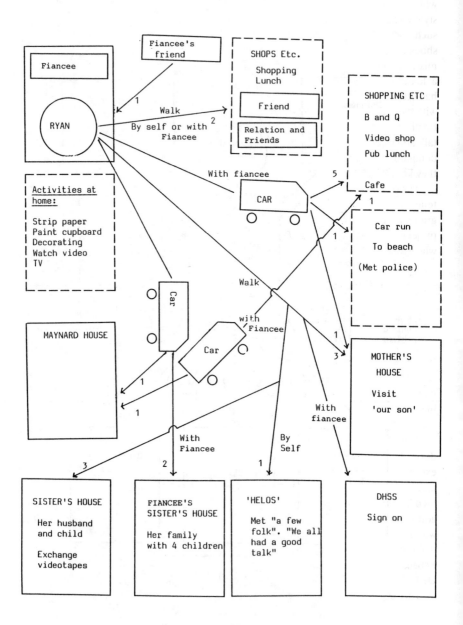

Fig. 2 - A week in the life of Ryan

which was unheard of at the time they began to inject drugs. To maintain their drug life-style Ryan and Dianne had to resort to shoplifting and house breaking. This reached such a level that they quickly became banned from city centre stores where suits and shoes to the value of £180 were being taken daily and resold for £50. By his own admission Ryan became well known to the police and to the courts and he reckons he has at least 'six-to-seven pages of previous convictions'. Detention centre and spells in prison had little effect on Ryan until the sombre reality of his and Dianne's HIV status, together with the realisation that James and their future together was more important than drugs, finally convinced them of the need to face up to their addiction. Ryan finds it hard to talk about his seropositivity and Dianne tends to deny the implications of her lympha-denopathy and weight loss. Both have a naive faith that everything will turn out right if they keep off drugs.

The court, in recognising the will for change, finally agreed in 1988 to a deferred sentence in respect of Ryan's latest offence provided he conform to a detoxification programme and attend Maynard House for counselling. A contract was drawn up by the project leader and agreed by Ryan, Dianne, Ryan's doctor and the project worker, Susan, who was going to undertake the counselling. The focus for Ryan's attendance would be:

- relapse prevention
- prevention of offending
- examination of coping methods and development of skills
- exploration of the relationship between Ryan and Dianne
- health issues and detoxification

It was furthermore agreed that Ryan would pick up his tablets (Dihydrocodeine (DF118s) and Diazepam around which the detoxification programme is built) on a fort-nightly basis. Sanctions would be considered if he started to inject again or sold his tablets to other users. Ryan was to see his doctor weekly for the doctor to monitor progress and HIV health.

During the period the researcher had contact with Ryan and Maynard House, Ryan's deferred sentence came up for review and was renewed for a further four months. Ryan expressed his wish to the researcher to remain in contact with Maynard House on a voluntary basis once this period of four months has been completed. He stated that he valued Susan's support and saw it as important that he and Dianne show her that they are getting to grips with their lives and are able to care for James. Ryan is progressing well with his detoxification programme and from a regime of 140 DF118s in October 1988 had reduced by February 1989 to 35 per week. He hopes to be drug free by the end of February 1989. Dianne (who thinks that Ryan is coming off too quickly) is still on 140 DF118s per week.

An examination of Ryan's networking reveals the importance of his social networks, his health networks, and his other support systems.

Social networks

Ryan's social networks can be divided up into family networks (his and Dianne's) and his friendship networks. The most important place for Ryan and Dianne is his mother's house and *Figure 2* shows that he visited there three times in the first monitored week. Often he visits daily to see 'our son'. Ryan talks of his little boy with considerable pride although James was born with mild cerebral palsy and has recently been in hospital for the insertion of grommets. Ryan does not find it easy to focus on his child's medical difficulties, especially his HIV status. Perhaps for Ryan and Dianne this is too much of a painful reminder of their own seropositivity. Ryan expresses great relief that his child is now no longer testing antibody positive and is cared for by his mum until 'we can take over the care'. Being with 'our son' is emotionally uplifting for Ryan and gives him a chance to feed and change the baby's nappies and show that he is capable of being a responsible and reliable father. Ryan's mother lives three minutes' away so access is easy by car or by walking. Ryan's older brother also lives with parents. Ryan also has two sisters living nearby both of whom he sees regularly and with one of whom he swaps video tapes. Dianne's sister and husband and four children are also visited regularly by car and provide Dianne with invaluable support. During the period the researcher was in contact with Ryan, Dianne fell out with her sister and relationships became very strained. Ryan would not discuss the reason except to say it was a 'domestic hassle and no loss to me'. This apparently is a regular occurrence for as Ryan put it, 'they are always falling out but they will start speaking again'. The family networks for Ryan and Dianne are shown in *Figure 3*.

The absence of Dianne's parental family suggests ambivalence about their daughter's former lifestyle and relationship with Ryan.

The most important factor in Ryan's own social network is his 'best friend' and his friend's fiancée. They live on the same estate as Ryan and Dianne, and are ex-drug users who are also coming off drugs. They were integral to the former drug using network of Ryan and Dianne and shared drugs and 'works' (drug injecting equipment) with them. It is not, therefore, surprising to know that both the best friend and his fiancée are also HIV positive. The shared drug using experiences and the HIV status have produced a strong bond between the two families.

First monitored week

Ryan's first monitored week, based on his diary, is shown in *Figure 2*. Like Ryan, his friend is also 'doing up' his flat and the consequence is that there is a lot of sharing of experiences and decorating resources between the two families. The commonalities of their former drug using lifestyles are now replaced by shared visits to the shops and to the pub. Ryan's friend is also a car driver whereas Ryan only has a provisional driving licence. Ryan relies on his friend accompanying him on longer car journeys, yet Ryan does not see this as necessary for shorter local journeys to the shops, rating the chances

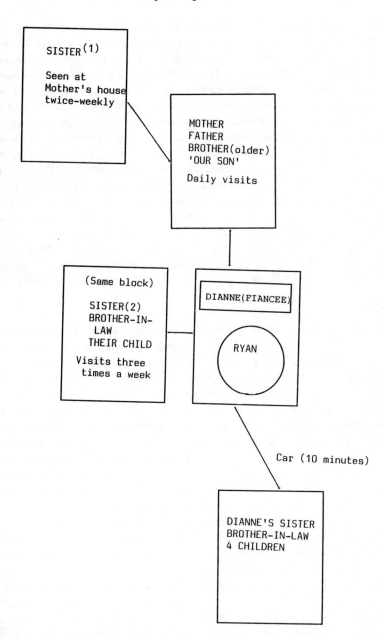

Fig. 3 - Family networks for Ryan and Dianne (fiancée)

of getting stopped by the police as minimal. The logic of this is interesting bearing in mind Ryan's desire to prove himself drug free and 'out of trouble' with the law. *Figure 2* shows him as having a drive one day in which they 'met police'. This was a drive to a local beauty spot three miles away and part of the object of outing was to give Dianne a driving lesson. Ryan's friend was accompanying them and the sighting of a car in which there were three known drug users obviously roused the curiosity of the local police. A police car travelling in the opposite direction turned and followed them, the outcome being that the car was stopped and as Ryan had no driving documents or insurance on him he was given five days to produce these at the local station. This incident highlights the need and value of assessing 'offender networks' in any analysis. Key figures in these networks for drug users could be probation officers, social workers, courts (District, County, High, etc.), chance encounters with local police, visits to solicitors and so forth.

Ryan's encounter with the police is illustrative of the difficulty many drug users have in 'going straight'. Their very presence on the street (or, as in Ryan's case in a car) can give rise to suspicion that an offence (drug deal) had been or was about to be committed. Further evidence of Ryan's difficulty in shaking off the offender label was illustrated by being recently stopped in the city centre on suspicion that he had been shoplifting again.

Health networks

The key person in Ryan's health network is undoubtedly his doctor. The particular group practice that Ryan attends is very experienced in dealing with drug users from the local area because of the high number and the fact that many are HIV positive. The particular group practice works closely with nurses, social workers, community psychiatrists, psychologists, drug projects and drug treatment clinics in producing an overall package of treatment care for individual patients. The ethos of this practice follows very much that laid down in 'Guidelines of Good Clinical Practice in the Treatment of Drug Misuse' (1984), namely that treatment of a drug user such as Ryan should be all-encompassing, not limited to the prescription of a substitute drug of dependence such as DF118. As has been already outlined, Ryan and his doctor are very much a part of the treatment contract, so that there is a clear awareness of the expectations of each other. Ryan sees his doctor weekly as part of the process of monitoring the withdrawal schedule and receives any health counselling and urine testing, etc., at that time. This process of monitoring is clearly important where HIV positivity is an added complication to the drug misuse for it is recognised that injudicious use of drugs will further compromise an immune system that is under stress from the virus.

Ryan speaks very well of his doctor, describing him as 'one of the best doctors I have ever met' and as a man who is 'interested in me'. The fifteen minute consultation is a highlight in Ryan's week. He takes great comfort in the doctor's assessment that 'his blood count is obviously good because of the spells spent in prison'. The doctor's report for Ryan's deferred sentence court appearance was seen by Ryan as being crucial. He described to the researcher that the doctor was 'delighted at his progress', that the doctor had described him in the report as 'a reliable patient that did not miss an appointment' and more importantly that 'Dianne was 90% better when Ryan was living with her than when he was in prison'. The doctor is also seen as important in giving Ryan advice about how to live well with HIV, especially over aspects of diet (Ryan is on a preferred high-fibre diet).

Supervision

Ryan's network shows the importance of two drug agencies in his weekly life, Helos and Maynard House.

Helos is a shop front drug project in the middle of the estate in which Ryan lives. Because of the many drug users that live in the locality Helos performs a very important function in providing a social outlet by which people with a drug problem can drop in and chat to the workers or share a coffee or game of pool or darts with anyone else who happens to be in the project. Helos, whilst not encouraging drug use on its premises also provides an important sanctuary for someone who has just used and needs help and support in what can best be described as 'a critical incident'. The project leader of Helos has known Ryan for some considerable time and he values the opportunity to drop in and see her or one of the workers for some advice. This service complements the more structured involvement of Maynard House and is recognised by all parties concerned. As Helos is a stone's throw from the group practice, links between the drug users, the project workers, and the general practitioners have been maximised to the benefit of all parties. Ryan and his best friend regularly drop in to Helos for a 'coffee and chat', a game of pool, and the centre now provides Ryan with the opportunity to participate regularly in five-a-side football. *Figure 2* shows this contact in the week in question.

Ryan attends for an appointment with Susan at Maynard House twice per week. By agreement he is often accompanied by Dianne. Despite the financial cost Ryan often travels to Maynard House by taxi because he says he gets 'bored on the bus'. Ryan sees Susan (his worker) as someone who will:

- help him with his drug problems
- help him with his domestic problems
- help him with his relationship with Dianne
- help him 'get back' James when the child is five

Despite the fact that Ryan didn't feel that the project had put into the court a 'good report about him because he has missed two appointments' he obviously sees attendance at the project as the main means of 'proving himself' and ultimately caring for his son.

In discussion with Susan, the researcher perceived her goals as follows:

- helping Ryan and Dianne to make decisions about their lives
- helping Ryan understand why he reacts the way he has done (highlighting the factors which could lead him to 'screw up his chances' or not)

- help Ryan work through his relationships

If there were any tensions the researcher saw these as relating to Ryan's need for Susan 'to put a good report in about him to the court' and to 'help him get his son back', of which neither goal was shared by Susan. A tension existed in that Ryan and Dianne tended to see Susan as someone who could make suggestions and give recommendations and advice, whilst Susan's approach was more reflective, aimed at enhancing Ryan's and Dianne's understanding of their social and drug using situation and thereby enabling them to make decisions.

Ryan gave the researcher the impression that he saw Susan as an important bridge between Dianne, himself and the statutory social worker who supervised James. Neither he nor Dianne felt that the social worker (whom they stated they didn't like) wanted them to care for James and therefore reports from the doctor and Susan on their progress would be needed to convince the court that they deserved to have the care of their child. The researcher felt that Susan did not want to get drawn into that debate.

Points for discussion

1. Assess the strengths and weaknessess of the different support systems of Ryan and Dianne as described. What are the implications for the formulation of social work plans and their implementation?
2. Comment on the differences of perspective between Ryan and Susan (the project worker from Maynard House) in relation to the drawing up of a contract.
3. Ryan's diary shows that he and Dianne have a high degree of mutual interdependence. This is born out by the fact that in seven years they have shared a lot, i.e.:
   - their relationship
   - friends
   - drugs and injecting equipment
   - the legal consequences of drug use
   - HIV
   - James

From what we know now:
   (a) How would Ryan cope if Dianne became progressively more ill?
   (b) How would Ryan cope if Dianne were unable to be drug free or if she were to relapse?

4. To what extent should Maynard House or the doctor tackle the denial Ryan and Dianne are showing to being HIV positive?
5. To what extent might Ryan's friend's HIV positivity influence future developments?

6. What are the long term objectives for James's care? Are Ryan and Dianne ever likely to care for their son? (If not, should the professionals be honest with them now and deal with any anger or drug relapse that may result?)

7. Ryan's mother features prominently in the care of 'our son'. How might she view the prospect of giving up the care of the child, especially as the child may have some handicap irrespective of the uncertainty of his HIV anti-body status?

8. What supports do Ryan's parents need? Who helps them reflect back over their son's drug career and if they experience guilt, anger over their son's and grandson's HIV status, who helps them with these feelings?

9. What, if any, specific knowledge and skill does a worker such as Susan need?

Matthew

Matthew (aged 26) has been married to Alison for three years and their first baby is expected in March 1989. They live in a one-bedroom privately rented flat about 15 minutes walk from Maynard House.

Matthew has been using drugs since he was a teenager. Smoking and cannabis were quickly replaced by heroin taken by intravenous injection. When heroin was not available he used Diconal in preference. Matthew has experimented with injecting Temgesics but does not prefer them as he says they do little for him. All in all, Matthew has been injecting and on occasions sharing 'equipment' for the last eight years. He has been tested several times for HIV and these tests have so far proved negative but he is described as being 'very worried about the disease'. Alison (who does not inject) has been tested for HIV and is also antibody negative. Matthew was referred to Maynard House in 1988 for counselling by a community psychiatrist to whom he had been referred by the general practitioner and hospital for advice about his drug use. Concern had been felt over Matthew's general state of health because since childhood he has had repeated problems with a collapsed lung and since he began injecting drugs he has had several admissions to hospital when the lung became filled with blood and fluid. The community psychiatrist had, therefore, placed Matthew on a treatment regime of oral Methadone by reduction in an attempt to stabilise his health and enable detoxification to be completed by early 1989. Both network drawings for the two monitored weeks based on diaries (*Figures 4* and *5*) show Matthew's visits to the doctor and then to the chemist to collect his Methadone.

Matthew's health network (see *Figure 6*) is fairly extensive and not untypical for a drug user in his position. The responsibilities added by his wife's health and pregnancy should also be noted.

As can been seen, the role of the General Practitioner is important as a key linkperson in Matthew's health care and the general care required by Alison. To this network will shortly be added the involvement of midwife and health visitor.

Matthew's health and his drug use are inextricably linked and are key factors in any assessment of how able he will be to stand up to the pressures of being a father. Already major concerns have been voiced by the community psychiatrist and Helen, his counsellor at Maynard House. These were put to the researcher as follows:

> Matthew is not looking well. Normally a drug user's health will improve when put on a Methadone maintenance regime but Matthew does not appear to be stabilising and is looking thinner and jaundiced. Matthew is complaining furthermore that the Methadone is making him sick (a recognised side effect). Is, therefore, Matthew taking his Methadone or is he selling it to other users in return for synthetic opiates and/or cannabis?

These concerns and others were shared with Matthew in counselling at the beginning of the period that the researcher was in contact with Maynard House. The following are Helen's brief notes for the researcher in that period:

> **Monday** - Joint meeting with Dr. T (community psychiatrist) and Matthew *re* reduction. Suspicions about selling and/or using other stuff voiced. M very defensive before this. Looked at the process of the interview - 'little boy lost routine'. M's feelings very closed but willing to work on this though finding it hard. Lot of mixed messages! Due in Wednesday.

> **Wednesday** - M phoned. Had been to hospital with wife. Had to go to GP to pick up results of some tests. Wouldn't be able to make it. Made appointment for Friday.

> **Friday** - M in. Feelings about last meeting explored. Where do we go from here? Concerns expressed about M's health particularly HIV. Housing issues explored - getting out of present area (family, relationships, future, where going, who M is, what he wants?) Responsibility issues are very convenient for M in present role. Agreed upon work to make sense of past. M to write down for the next meeting his perceptions of himself. Agreed to work with Alison every third meeting.

Three months later a significant pattern of events was reported by Helen to the researcher which appeared to lend weight to the concerns that she and the community psychiatrist had previously expressed.

1. Although Matthew kept diaries for two separate periods for the researcher, his attendance at Maynard House tailed off abruptly from twice per week to once every six weeks or longer. Appointments were not kept and (unlike previously) no phone contact was made to change appointments. When eventually seen Matthew said he 'had lost interest in coming to the project' and used his wife's pregnancy and her hospital ante-natal appointments as a reason also for not coming to Maynard House.

2. Initially when Alison had come for a joint meeting with her husband and Helen, her openness and frankness was noted to be in marked contrast to Matthew and it was clear that he was embarrassed by her revelations. Subsequently Matthew has fended off contact between Maynard House and his wife.

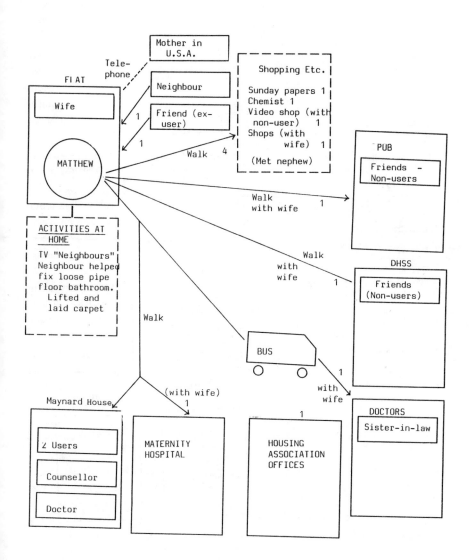

Fig. 4 - A week in Matthew's life (first monitored period)

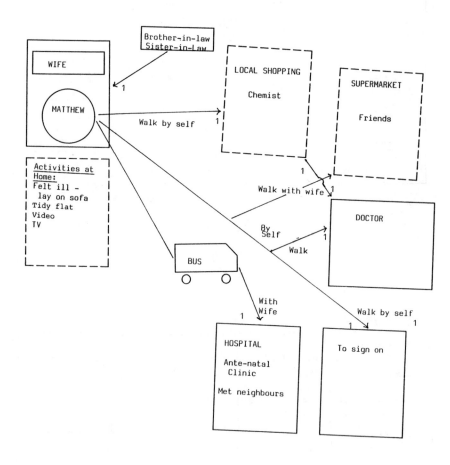

Fig. 5 - A week in Matthew's life (second monitored period)

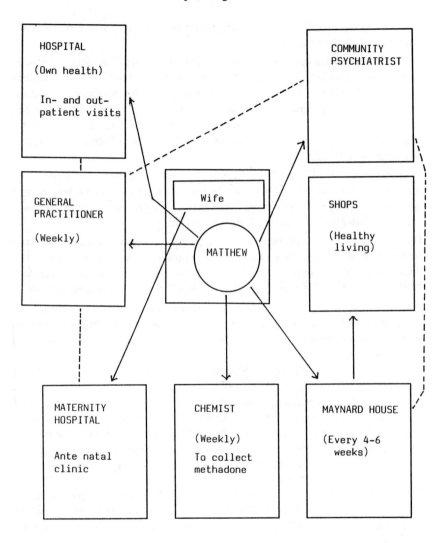

HOSPITAL

(Own health)

In- and out-patient visits

GENERAL PRACTITIONER

(Weekly)

Wife

MATTHEW

COMMUNITY PSYCHIATRIST

SHOPS

(Healthy living)

MATERNITY HOSPITAL

Ante natal clinic

CHEMIST

(Weekly)

To collect methadone

MAYNARD HOUSE

(Every 4-6 weeks)

Key: _____Client contact

    ---------Joint meetings

Fig. 6 - Matthew's health support network

3. In a joint interview Alison reported to Helen that she had had to send drug users who were hanging around the house 'packing'.

4. The police raided Matthew and Alison's flat and found a small quantity of cannabis and a spoon (possibly for mixing drugs). Alison admitted smoking 'hash'. Matthew claims that they were 'set up by the police' but he seemed remarkably vague and ambivalent about making contact with a lawyer to discuss their defence. The court case is pending. The police action was described as a 'big raid' in which 'their door was kicked down' and left the counsellor wondering if Matthew had been tipped off as so few drugs were found.

5. Matthew was involved in a fight in which he claimed he was mugged by an unknown assailant. He had to be admitted to 'accident and emergency' at a local hospital with a cracked cheekbone. Was he mugged or was this a drug related assault? The assailant was not identified. Therefore there were no charges.

6. Other workers in the project report that their clients from other parts of the city know of Matthew 'on the grape vine'. These clients are often much younger or older established users who do not live in Matthew's neighbourhood. The uncomfortable feeling has been left that Matthew's flat (if not himself) is a centre for drug dealing.

The researcher was not able to meet Matthew. An appointment had to be cancelled because of Matthew and Alison's delay at the maternity hospital. Matthew said to the researcher 'Do you really want to see me?' An appointment was made for the following day which was not kept.

Matthew is an only son. He has only fleeting contact with his father who lives thirty miles away. Matthew's parents split up when he was 14. His mother lives in America and he has weekly contact with her by phone. Matthew's mother has sent him money regularly despite the fact that in the early days she was aware that it might be spent on drugs. Matthew initially trained as a pipe welder and for four years the money from his trade together with the money from his mother ensured that (a) his drug supply was paid for and (b) his involvement with the police was peripheral, involving one incident of possession of cannabis for personal use.

Alison's parents live outside the city and are in regular contact. Matthew's father-in-law (who runs a coal business) offered his son-in-law a job and accommodation but Matthew turned this offer down. Would such a move have taken Matthew an unacceptable distance away from his drug using network?

Figure 5 shows contact with his brother and sister-in-law (and nephew). The brother-in-law is an 'ex-user'.

Housing is an important issue for Matthew and Alison and is reflected in their network. *Figure 4* shows a visit to the Housing Association and Matthew's skills and trade came in handy for dealing with a D.I.Y. problem in the house during Week One:

'Had loose pipe in toilet, bathroom flooded.

Fixed pipe with help of neighbour.

Lifted carpet in toilet to dry.

Layed carpet in toilet.'

Their present flat is cramped and inadequate for a couple expecting their first baby. It is in need of major improvements. It is privately rented. Security of tenure is guaranteed by the DHSS payment but Matthew and Alison hope that the housing association will find them something more suitable. (Housing associations have turned out to be major saviour of couples like Matthew and Alison who require good standard low cost housing. They also have the potential for more innovative forms of referral and nomination thereby making it possible for drug users and people with HIV or AIDS to gain access to the local housing stock without discrimination.) The dilemma for Matthew is that much of the 'hard to let' property is in areas of the city where there is not only active drug use but also a known substantial spread of HIV among the drug using community. For someone who is trying to come off drugs and support a wife and a new baby at the same time this would pose considerable difficulties. The tension for Matthew is whether he has a commitment to break with his drug using network. Already he has rejected an offer to move out of this area and it is very arguable that for him there may well be important reasons for staying in his present area.

Matthew's diary for the first week shows that most of his world seems to be divided up into users, non users, and ex-users (the exception being a neighbour and a cousin). Just as Maynard House has doubts as to whether Matthew is coming off drugs, so he, also, has doubts as to whether some of his friends are really off drugs. The division of acquaintances and friends, according to whether they are, or are not, part of the drugs scene, is a major task for people like Matthew. The social norms of friendship are compounded by such issues as:

- is this person a user, ex-user?
- will this person offer me drugs and how will I react?
- does this person want drugs, know my reputation and expect me to carry drugs which they can offer to buy?
- what risk (if any) does this person pose to me in respect of hepatitis B or HIV?
- what other risks, (assault, police involvement, informing) does this person pose?

Matthew's diary is illustrative of someone sorting out his social situation and their friendship boundaries.

Week 1, day 2 - 'Went to pub with wife and a couple of friends (non users). Met a few pub regulars - no one I have known in the past, just locals that I know to acknowledge.'

Week 1, day 4 - 'Visit to Maynard House met counsellor, doctor and "two users".'

Week 1, day 5 - a.m. 'To DHSS to sign on. Met two casual acquaintances, two so-called "ex users".'

Week 1, day 5 - p.m. 'Boring. Stayed in all afternoon and watched videos. Smoked mackeral for late tea. Friend "ex-user" came to visit.'

The diary for Week 2 (*Figure 5*) shows less of an overt preoccupation with the drug world, more staying in with his wife and much more walking by himself to supermarkets, shops, and the DHSS as Alison progresses further into her pregnancy.

It is difficult for Helen and Maynard House to assess Matthew's parenthood skills. At present he is being a dutiful father accompanying his wife to maternity hospital. However, when he is seen, he presents to his counsellor as daunted and yet excited by the birth of the baby. He wavers between concern for Alison and concern for the baby seeing the birth as a reason for him 'settling down and accepting responsibility'. The experience of many drug workers has been that drug users can make very good parents. It is unhelpful to label people like Matthew as 'chaotic' and 'irresponsible' and unable to provide the care required for a child. Sometimes it can help in that they are seen as being in a sense 'on trial'.

The main concern is whether the responsibility will be too much for Matthew. Will he seek solace in more visits to the pub or more use of drugs? Matthew's counsellor expressed her concerns to the researcher in wondering whether Matthew would 'do a bunk' when the baby is born.

Alison has always been seen as the more powerful, honest and 'up front' person of the couple. She is being shielded from contact with Maynard House. When the baby is born she may be less able to monitor Matthew's drug use, his contact with drug using friends, or limit any dealing that may be going on. It will not be helpful for Alison to have two people dependent on her - Matthew and the baby. If Matthew does not provide the support there may well be an increased involvement in the family life of her parents, her sister and brother.

Points for discussion

1. How justified is the concern about whether Matthew and Alison will face up to their future responsibilities?

2. How will Matthew cope? Will he feel pushed out by the baby and his wife's family and, if so, will he relapse into his former state of drug use?

3. Given Matthew's withdrawal from regular contact with Maynard House, where is the most appropriate point for safer sex and safer drug use counselling for him?

4. Given Matthew's ambivalence about his contact with Maynard House, what would be his reaction if his case were to be closed? Where would such a decision leave Alison?

5. What are the next stages for Matthew's detoxification programme? Review? New detoxification goal? Maintenance on safer drug use through longer term prescribing of opiate substitute other than methadone?

6. To what extent (if any) will the impending court case for possession of cannabis be likely to shape events for Matthew and Alison?

7. Discuss the effects of the housing problem on Matthew and Alison's situation.

8. Discuss Matthew's tendency to describe his friends and acquaintances in terms of whether they are drug users or ex-users or non-users.

Richard

Richard (aged 27) lives with his parents in their three bedroom flat about three miles from Maynard House. He presents as a bright alert young man and has been attending Maynard House for the last six months where his counsellor, Jean, is the senior project worker. He is highly motivated to counselling and, since his detoxification, has become a regular member of Alcoholics and Narcotics Anonymous groups in the city. Richard's drug history prior to his 'reformation' (as he sees it) shows a considerable and varied use of drugs. This is summarised as follows:

At school. Used amphetamines recreationally whilst still at school. The euphoria, increased alertness, increased self esteem and self confidence helped a very active teenager who (although 'he knew it was wrong') found the drug very beneficial to the 'all night dancing cult at weekends'.

Aged 18. After two years on 'uppers' started using barbiturates (Seconal, Tuinal, Mandrax) and found barbiturates and alcohol 'a real party piece for a while'. Richard lived in an area where chemist's shops were regularly being broken into and as he was, in his terms, 'close to the source', the availability and the low price meant that he quickly became a drug dependent. Richard's cousin died of a 'downer's overdose' at this time but whilst he admits that it should have made a difference to his own drug use it did not. Richard's drug use rapidly became more varied with regular use of cannabis, diazepam (Valium) and alcohol being the preferred drugs of choice.

Aged 21. Richard discovered heroin and other opiate drugs (Diconal, Palfium, Pethidine). He began sporadically to inject but was still working and felt 'in control'.

Aged 23. 'Smoking and snorting' - 'anything that went up my nose and down my throat'. Richard was now using Dihydrocodeine (DF118s) and physeptone (Methadone linctus or mixture) in preference.

Aged 25. By chance discovered codeine linctus. He graphically describes his reaction to the opiate feeling as 'Christ what's this. It's like happy birthday'. He drank half the bottle! Richard quickly became addicted to the linctus and on moving to the

London area found it much more easily available than in his home town. Richard stated also that he tried cocaine three times and LSD seven times.

Aged 25-27. Tried to come off codeine linctus but whilst withdrawing he upped his alcohol consumption considerably (two bottles of brandy a day). Realising that he had to do something as he was feeling his life was getting out of control, he left London, returned home and sought help from his G.P. He was referred to a psychiatrist for help through hospital outpatient detoxification and having heard of Maynard House through a friend sought help and counselling from them as well.

Richard has shared injecting equipment in the past but reckons that this was before HIV 'was around'. He has not been tested for HIV but does not find it easy to discuss the subject. The researcher (who met Richard twice) felt that there were nagging doubts in the back of his mind but that he preferred not to know his sero-status.

Richard managed to fund his drug habit over the years because he served an apprenticeship and then became 'time served' in a skilled trade. By the age of 23 he reckoned he was clearing £220 a week and his drug use escalated when he received several thousands of pounds redundancy money. Although currently unemployed Richard is helping out at an art restorer's and is actively seeking re-employment in his former trade.

Drugs, and particularly alcohol, have played a very important role in shaping Richard's family relationships, both when he was using drugs and now that he is being treated.

- Richard's father works in a local brewery.
- a cousin has died from a drug overdose.
- a cousin has had drug problems and attends Narcotics Anonymous.
- an aunt attends Al-Anon (a support group for relatives of people with an alcohol problem).

Home life stability is often determined by how much alcohol Richard's father has consumed at work or after work. Richard admits to be being edgy in his father's company when his father drinks and, although he accepted his son's sobriety, father and son do not appear to have a close relationship. Richard describes his mother (a personal assistant to a shipping company executive) as having had a 'blind spot' for him whilst he was taking drugs. Now he feels they could not have a better relationship as 'I do not have to hide anything any more'.

Christmas and New Year were difficult periods for Richard in his new found sobriety. The support of the AA and NA groups were crucial. The anticipation of what would go wrong was, he felt, ten times worse than what happened. The effect on his social networks was interesting:

1. Increased attendance at NA and AA support meetings.

2. Some family functions not attended. As Richard described it to the researcher; 'Not that I did not want to participate, rather I did not want to put myself in difficult or uncomfortable situations.'

3. 'Not running around the family houses like I used to do.'

Not all Richard's extended family know of his sobriety, so rather than 'mentally cataloging excuses' for not attending certain functions he had to devise mechanisms so that people assumed he was drinking a mixer containing alcohol. ('Coca Cola came in very handy!')

The first monitored week of Richard's activities (*Figure 7*) shows clearly his reliance on AA and NA support meetings and being in the company of their members.

Day 1. Coffee with AA member

Day 1. Evening AA meeting

Day 2. Evening visit to NA member at his home (cousin ex-user)

Day 3. Lunch time AA meeting

Day 3. Evening AA meeting

Day 4. Evening NA meeting

Day 5. Evening AA meeting

Day 6. Evening AA meeting

The second monitored week (*Figure 8*) shows a similar heavy reliance on the support framework provided by NA and AA.

Richard has wholeheartedly embraced the philosophy of AA and NA. He describes himself to the researcher as a 'Junkie without the Junk'.

He sees himself as at very early recovery stage of an illness/disease that will take a lifetime to come to terms with. Richard's friendship patterns are also very much dictated by those contacts he makes at NA and AA. He sees the people who attend these meetings as 'winners' and it is indicative that he said to the researcher:

'I'll pick my friends, I'll pick the winners.'

Richard feels comfortable with the support framework provided by NA and AA and believes fervently that 'if it is correct it will work for you'.

Richard's first monitored week (*Figure 7*) shows that, on the whole, he kept himself to himself. He journeyed mainly by himself and his visits were 'functional' rather than purely social, i.e. to various agencies or groups. The first week does, however, show Richard attending a funeral of an ex-girlfriend's father. Richard is very much at the sexual crossroads at the moment. He would like to get married one day but is deliberately holding himself back from establishing new relationships until he has sorted himself out. He told the researcher that he did not want to get drawn into a new relationship at present as:

'I need to learn about myself before learning about someone else.'

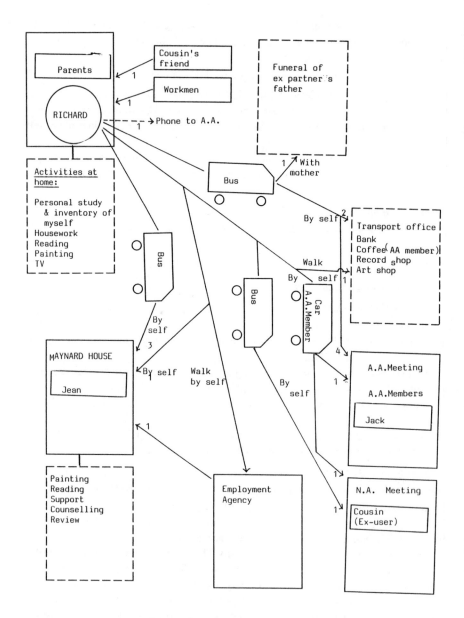

Fig. 7 - A week in Richard's life (first monitored period)

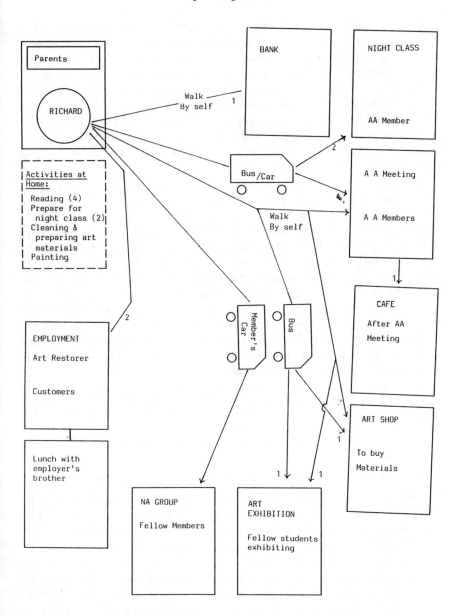

Fig. 8 - A week in Richard's life (second monitored period)

Richard's previous relationships have been longstanding and intense. He felt that he had to attend the funeral of his ex-girlfriend's father because the latter had been good to him. Despite the fact that the girlfriend has married and that it might have been painful for Richard to attend the funeral (meeting her and her husband as he did) he still went. Richard has, however, not totally submerged his sexual sparkle! He described to the researcher with avidness that whilst waiting for their second meeting he had coincidentally met a female visitor (not client) in the reception area of Maynard House. He mentally set himself the task of getting this lady's name and address under some pretext because 'I fancied her and I wanted to see if I still had what it takes'. He achieved his goal before seeing the researcher!

Richard's contact with Maynard House and Jean (his counsellor) is much more intense in the first week (*Figure 7*) than in the second week (*Figure 8*). This reflects the use he has made of Maynard House, not only for counselling (once per week) but also for taking advantage of their recreational facilities for drug users. It was through the use of one primary facility, the Art room, that it quickly became apparent that Richard has the potential for being a very talented artist. That this talent is beginning to be realised, can be seen in Week Two of the diary, as Richard is seen now working part-time with an art restorer. He is also painting, and attending art school at nights and subsequent exhibitions. Developing this talent has been a major breakthrough for Richard and is indicative of the role and value diversional activities can play for some ex-drug users.

Richard describes himself as easily bored. Art therapy undoubtedly has alleviated much of this boredom. Art for Richard has also meant exploring new dimensions and taking risks. He described this to the researcher:

'I feel I am more expressive and confident in my painting. I only used to play with safe areas, figures in the distance. Now I can paint people more close up and more distinctive'.

Richard sees links between his AA 'treatment' and his art. He described this to the researcher thus:

'I need the meetings to help me understand myself, then I can paint.'

The therapeutic value of painting at Maynard House has enabled Richard to open up part of his personality which, like his drug abuse, were very personal and locked away. Jean has been able to develop and use this experience as part of counselling and both she and Richard have recognised that while art can unlock his feelings it could also have the potential for camouflaging his feelings.

Now that Richard has been able to develop his artistic interests there has been achieved a more balanced focus to his life. This is reflected in Week Two (*Figure 8*) where the focus is less on 'help' contacts than in Week One (*Figure 7*). There is as a result an air of greater confidence about the network!

Richard values very much his contact with Maynard House and the affirmation he has received from Jean his counsellor. He describes Jean as 'knowing what I am thinking before I know it.' Counselling has helped Richard (in his own words) to 'Discover that I do have the power of choice.'

From Jean's perspective counselling goals are:

- helping Richard make sense of life at home.
- helping Richard make sense of past drug experiences.
- helping Richard manage stresses.
- giving space for Richard to check out what has been happening to him in the past week and identify issues that are around which need working on.

Longer-term goals are to work on the areas of 'self-pity' and allow Richard to express strong feelings. Richard will need help also in determining longer term relationships, employment and accommodation goals.

Jean has also raised the question of HIV and safer sex practices. Richard has not, it appears, found it easy to take either on board in counselling although he is conscious of the health issues and sees his doctor once per month, not only to obtain his sickness certificate, but also for discussion about diet and healthy eating. Richard is, however, still a smoker.

Richard's support network is illustrated in *Figure 9*.

Points for discussion

1. How able is Richard to integrate the changes that are happening in his life to nuclear and extended family relationships?

2. To what extent (if any) does Richard's adherence to the sick/disease role 'junkie/alcoholic' label inhibit his future opportunities and the development of his networks?

3. Life is very 'comfortable' for Richard at the moment. To what extent is there a denial of real feelings of anger and frustration at his drug using past? Are these feelings being suppressed in his art and attendance at AA - NA meetings? Should Jean consider more overtly 'rocking the boat' in counselling?

4. The issues around HIV are largely unresolved as are the issues around safer sex. To what extent, given what we know of Richard's past, should these be developed in counselling?

5. Richard's sexuality has to some extent become subliminal. To what extent should these feelings be worked on and what effect are they likely to have on his future networking patterns?

6. To what extent has Richard become dependent on home, AA - NA and Maynard House? How validated will he feel if he strikes out in new directions and tests himself out?

7. When (and if) Richard resumes his old trade, what effect will this (and the financial benefits) have on his networks and general lifestyle? If he is really good should Ri-

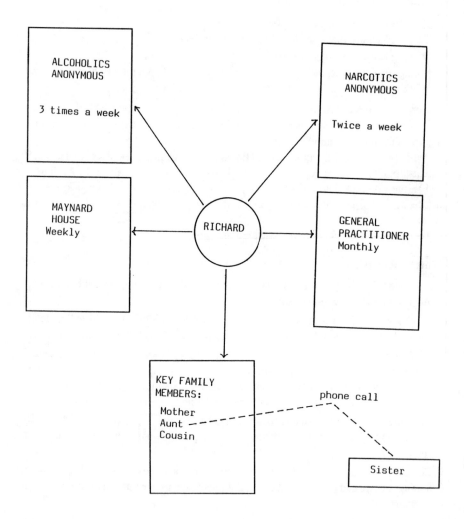

Fig. 9 - Illustration of Richard's support network

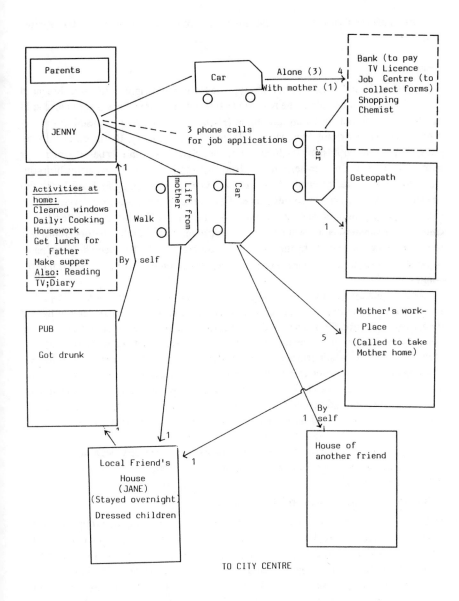

Parents

JENNY

Car   Alone (3)   4
       With mother (1)

Bank (to pay
   TV Licence
Job Centre (to
   collect forms)
Shopping
Chemist

3 phone calls
for job applications

Car

Osteopath

Activities at
home:
Cleaned windows
Daily: Cooking
Housework
Get lunch for
   Father
Make supper
Also: Reading
TV;Diary

Walk

Lift from
mother

Car

By) self

1

PUB

Got drunk

Mother's work-
   Place
(Called to take
Mother home)

5

By
self
1

1

1

Local Friend's
   House
   (JANE)
(Stayed overnight)
Dressed children

1

House of
another friend

TO CITY CENTRE

Fig. 10 - A week in Jenny's life (a) local network

chard abandon his former trade and aim for a career in art or an art-related occupation?

Jenny

Jenny is aged 31 and lives with her parents in a town about eight miles from Maynard House. The diary she kept for the researcher showed that her week was very much split up between activities based around home (*Figure 10*) and activities based in the city centre with her boyfriend Alan who is HIV positive (*Figure 11*). By the end of the researcher's contact with Jenny the focus for her activities was primarily based around her home. She had split up from her boyfriend having been instrumental in getting him convicted for drug-related offences. Alan is currently in prison awaiting trial and Jenny will be called as a key witness. In consequence, she is very afraid of going into the city in case she is recognised and 'done over' by any of Alan's friends. This crisis has affected her contact with Maynard House which is more peripheral to her life than before. Jenny was referred to Maynard House by the community psychiatrist who had been helping her to come off drugs and had initiated a reducing detoxification programme based on methadone.

Jenny began using drugs as a teenager when the crowd she went around with (which she describes as 'middle class and all with well off parents') began experimenting and then using recreationally a range of drugs including cannabis, amphetamines, cocaine, LSD. By her early twenties she had moved into a city centre flat and was a regular user of heroin (one-and-a-half grams per day) with a £150 a day habit. Jenny prides herself on being rarely unemployed and 'paying her way' when it came to drugs. She has worked as a local government clerical officer, civil servant, estate agent clerk, nursing auxilliary, care assistant in and old people's home and a nursing agency relief worker during this period. At the height of her heroin use Jenny supplemented her income by working as a sauna operative which was, in itself, a front for sex-industry work.

Throughout the last ten years, Jenny's networking has entirely been dominated by her own drug use and association with drug users. She described her friendship network to the researcher as:

'I didn't have any non-drug related friends'.

Jenny was, during this time, moving in and out of a small compact group of friends (users). She was using and dealing (buying and selling) whatever happened to be around. Jenny facilitated her drug availability in the past by seeing three doctors (a) at home (b) in the city and (c) in another town. All of them were unaware of each other's involvement. By this method, she obtained dihydrocodeine (DF118's) diazepam (Valium 10,5,2, mg. tablets) and temazepam with relative ease. Jenny described her use of drugs as 'sporadic' and claimed to the researcher that she was able to come off whenever she wanted.

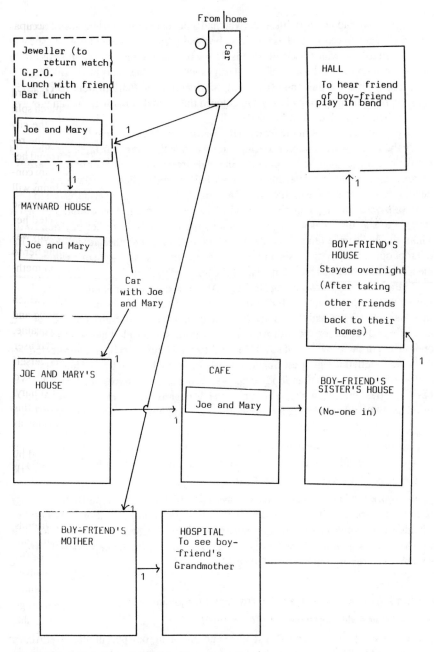

Fig. 11 - A week in Jenny's life (b) city centre network

Once Jenny had met up with Alan (who had a penchant for breaking into chemists) all this changed. Recreational use of drugs became regular dependent use and she was introduced to a far wider circle of friends. Jenny recalls that they had cupboards full of needles available in the boyfriend's flat. Drugs such as cocaine, morphine, codeine, diamorphine (heroin), dipipanone (Diconal), Methadone and Palfium were freely available. On reflection, although Jenny had enjoyed this period of her life, she can now say, 'God. When you look back, it was dreadful!'

Hepatitis B caused periodic scares. HIV was unknown at the time.

By the time she was 26 Jenny decided to try and make a break from drugs. She sold her flat and moved back to her parents. She had already lost a number of jobs because of her drug use and was determined to seek help as she wished to pursue a career in nursing. She came clean with the three General Practitioners and was referred to hospital for psychiatric help and detoxification. The period since has represented for her a struggle to stay off drugs while surrounded by the drug culture of her boyfriend with whom she had decided to remain. Jenny began to channel her energies into caring for other people recognising, as she put it, that she needed 'to have someone who needed me'. This 'someone' ranged from Alan to the hospital patients.

At the time Jenny was coming off drugs, Alan was diagnosed as being HIV positive. For Jenny the whole issue of AIDS came as a major shock. Not only had she been aware that Alan and friends had shared needles (she denies sharing herself), but she had had an active and varied sex life with Alan. Furthermore, she recalled her work as a sauna operative and the provision of sexual 'extras' to the clients. Oral and unprotected sex had always netted the greatest financial rewards. Jenny had the first of her HIV tests and was found to be HIV antibody negative. Repeated tests have shown that she has been negative since. How she has remained HIV negative she does not know. Alan refused to contemplate wearing a condom for sex saying that he didn't like them. Jenny put it thus to the researcher:

> 'He said he couldn't or wouldn't use a condom. He said he had no need for condoms and when he did try to use one (when he was not too stoned or drunk to have sex) he always lost his erection so we gave up.'

The network for Jenny's week is as we have said, divided into two parts, namely 'city centre activities' and 'home activities'. The intensity of Jenny's relationships with her friends is apparent from the city centre network (*Figure 11*). She throws herself into life with her friends. Extracts from her diary for Day 2, from which the network is drawn, illustrate the intensity and high level of activity:

Day 2

Morning - Got up at 8.30 a.m. To city centre for job interview.

Lunchtime - Met boyfriend in Cafe for lunch.

Afternoon - With boyfriend to post office and station for passport photos. Met Alan's
    mate at GPO. Then went to local bar for an orange juice with them. To Maynard

House for appointment with Jean (counsellor), met Joe and Mary, returned to the bar for a drink afterwards.

Evening - Went to Joe and Mary's house stayed there for two and a half hours. Went to boyfriend's sister's house 'no one in', went back to boyfriend's house, stayed there till 1.15 a.m., drove home to bed (2.05 a.m.)

When at home, Jenny is very active in caring for her parents. (See *Figure 10*.) She is very energetic at home - her diary gives her getting up early each day and illustrates that she can have a late night and still be up early the next day. The intensity of her activity at home is also illustrated in Jenny's diary:

Day 1

Morning - Cleaned lounge windows, vacuumed lounge, washed kitchen floor, cleaned kitchen window, made lasagne for tea, got laundry ready for father.

Afternoon/evening - Tidied bedroom, collected mother from work, set table for tea, washed dishes, went to bed around midnight.

Day 2

Morning - Cleaned bedroom windows, did washing and ironing, prepared lunch.

Afternoon/evening - Collected mother from work, paid TV licence at bank, went to job centre, did shopping, made soup and quiche for tea, had tea, washed dishes, made rum punch for parents, went to bed 1 a.m.

Day 4

Morning - Got up late 11.30 a.m. (late night). Washed dishes, made lunch, vacuumed lounge, washed more dishes after lunch with father.

Afternoon/evening - Cleaned out wardrobe of summer clothes for storage, cleaned bathroom, collected prescription, took mother to osteopath, set table, made tea, washed dishes, to bed around midnight.

The diary illustrates Jenny's keenness to care for her parents and one wonders if there is an expiatory element in her behaviour, as now she relies heavily on them for support and admits she must have caused them considerable anxiety over the years with her drug use. Jenny describes her parents as standing by her. They know of her drug problems but she has only confided in her mother that she worked in a sauna parlour.

Jenny's social networks have been, to a large extent, dictated by her involvement with Alan. His flat became a base for her to stay but it also brought her into contact with drug users and drug dealers at a time when she was trying to sort herself out in respect to drugs. She describes the block of flats as being owned by a drug supplier and the control of lettings by a caretaker who was himself involved in drug dealing and who preferred to let to people 'on the scene'.

Jenny's diary shows the close involvement with boyfriend, his friends and his family. During the period under review she rapidly became disenchanted with both the drug scene and her boyfriend, feeling that their relationship was going nowhere. Jenny moved out of Alan's flat and obtained a flat of her own nearby. She also made an attempt to break off the relationship but came under considerable emotional pressure and blackmail from Alan who threatened to implicate her in the break-ins to chemists and subsequent drug using and dealing. During this period Alan broke into another chemist obtaining large quantities of temazepam and barbiturates. Alan's threats finally led to a showdown with Jenny in which he violently assaulted both her and her car and she decided enough was enough. Even though it meant putting herself on the line, Jenny went to the police and made a full statement implicating Alan, the caretaker, and a wide variety of drug dealers in a series of crimes. As a result of this and subsequent police raids, drug friends and dealers are in prison on remand awaiting trial. The resolution of this crisis has had a marked effect on a number of Jenny's networks.

Firstly, the crisis had an effect on the health networks. (See *Figure 12*.) Jenny's GP is playing a prominent role in supporting her with the emotional trauma resulting from the confession to the police and the subsequent trial. A psychiatrist is also providing background reports on Jenny for the trial and the prosecution legal team.

Secondly, the crisis had an effect on the legal network (see *Figure 13*). Solicitor A is dealing with the interdicts Jenny requires to protect herself from Alan and unwelcome intrusions from drug friends and associates. Solicitor B is dealing with the impending court case and briefing of barristers, etc. Solicitor C is dealing with the sale of Jenny's city flat and linking to Solicitor D, family solicitor.

Thirdly, the crisis has affected Jenny's social networks. Jenny very rarely comes into the city now for fear of being seen by drug users. Her pride and main means of transport had been a very distinctive 'Mini' car on which she had lavished a lot of attention. She is now selling the car because it is a threat to her desired anonymity. Jenny's social life is now entirely home-based. She did not keep a second diary for the researcher because of her total involvement in subsequent events and her fear of making any further disclosures about herself on paper. She did, however, agree to meet the researcher. From this meeting the researcher gained the information on which the current network (shown in *Figure 14*) is based. Jenny is now working in a restaurant, near her home, waitressing, doing some cooking and selling ice cream and cigarettes. Her local friend (see *Figure 10*) at whose house she had stayed and who had 'dressed children' is now playing a prominent role in her social networking. Jane is a friend from school days and has three children. She attends a post-natal group and Jenny has been babysitting for her and helps to take the children to church and Sunday school.

Jenny now has more contact with her sister and two brothers who live in a city about 150 miles away from her home. These links are seen as very important to Jenny for a variety of reasons:

1. A relative of her father has died and her flat is up for sale. Jenny is thinking about putting in a bid for it.

2. Jenny wants to move closer to her brothers and sister.

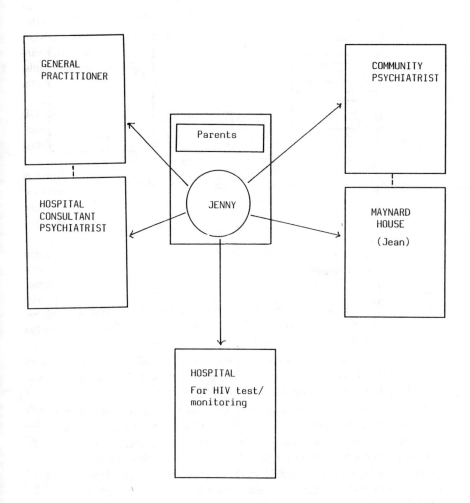

Fig. 12 - Jenny's health support network

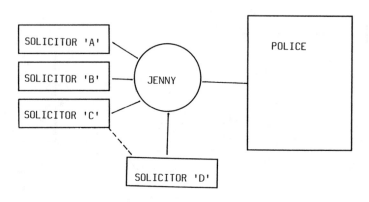

Fig. 13 - Jenny's legal network

3. Jenny is keen to train as a nurse. Although she began nurse training several years ago she discontinued the course. This city has an established college of nursing and Jenny is attracted by the possibility of training there.

4. The city has a relatively low known drug scene and HIV/AIDS statistics. Jenny feels 'safe' there. There is also a city based drug project at which she could obtain counselling if she felt she needed it.

Jenny comes across as an animated person with a high degree of nervous energy. She continues to make the most of every day saying she finds it 'hard if she is bored'. Jenny is struggling to maintain her contact with Maynard House at present but claims that she finds her contact with Jean helpful. The challenging approach of the community psychiatrist Jenny finds hard to handle. Jenny realises that she will need all the help she can get when the court case comes up especially as it will mean confronting her former boyfriend and doubtless being subjected to rigorous cross examination by his counsel. She expects a lot of 'drug dirty linen' to be washed in court and in consequence she does not want her father there. She is afraid of what might come out that he does not know about. Her GP has offered 'sedatives' if matters get too much to handle.

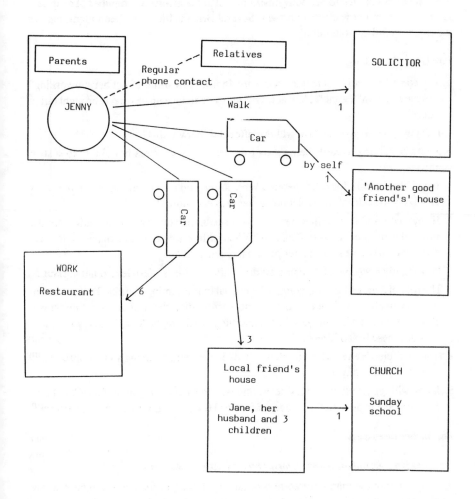

Fig. 14 - Jenny's current network

Jenny is afraid of Alan or 'drug heavies' (her words) finding her as a consequence of what she has done. Resolving the 'fight/flight' dilemma represents a major tension for Jenny. Part of her wants to fight the drug scene and come clean over her involvement with drugs (this has led to her being instrumental in the arrests of a number of drug dealers) and part of her wants to run away. Several British cities have been mentioned as places she could 'go to ground'.

Points for discussion

1. The court case will be a major trauma for Jenny. How will it affect her networking? (Social? Health? Legal?) How able will Jenny be to face up to what is brought out in court?

2. If Jenny 'goes to ground' how will this affect her networking?

3. Jenny is working towards being drug free. How do you assess her ability to sustain this?

4. Jenny likes to care for other people. Who, at the end of the day, cares for Jenny? Is she likely to seek solace in alcohol as her primary choice?

5. Jenny's counsellor describes her as a 'very sexual person'. Would you advocate the principles of safer sex and if so, how? What difference could this make to her lifestyle given what we know of her personality and past?

6. In what other ways would coming off drugs affect Jenny's lifestyle and networking?

7. The role of Jenny's family is going to be crucial in the coming months. To what extent are they likely to be influenced by events surrounding the trial and what effect will this have on Jenny's family? What counselling needs might Jenny's family have and how are these best addressed?

8. How can Jenny's energy best be channelled? Is a career in nursing an appropriate and realistic opportunity in this respect?

9. Jenny will require further HIV tests. She last had sex with Alan before Christmas. How will she cope with the anxiety of further HIV tests, as well as other pressures?

For further discussion

Men who have sex with men and women who have sex with women

A recognition of the inappropriateness of talking about 'gay men and women' and the 'gay community' is long overdue. The description 'men who have sex with men' now being used by the Health Education Authority in current HIV campaigns is perhaps a belated acknowledgement of the fact that gay and bisexual men and women do not fall into neatly identifiable categories either as individuals or social groupings. The targeting of this section of society for action, advice and education about HIV and AIDS has to be approached with care and a great deal of sensitivity. It is manifestly clear that HIV has been no respector of sexual identity. It is also important to recognise the diversity of social and sexual behaviours comprising the homosexual/bisexual experience. As a result, it is as equally misleading to describe the heterosexual experience as 'straight' and therefore, by definition, normative. This is to marginalise homosexual people 'by the use' of homophobically contrasting adjectives such as 'bent' or 'deviant'.

It is possibly, therefore, of more value to look at the impact of HIV on the social networking of men and women who have sex with a person of the same sex and to relate, in consequence, any safer sex education programmes. An innovative use of diaries as a way of evaluating networking and also as a way of providing a first hand database of the sexual activity and changing sexual behaviour of such men is currently being undertaken by 'Project Sigma' South Bank Polytechnic London. The broad aims of this three-year project are:

1. To investigate the inter-relationship between types and patterns of sexual behaviour and the presence of HIV antibodies.

2. To examine the sexual behaviour of gay men in relation to the progression to AIDS in those who are HIV positive.

3. To monitor changes in sexual behaviour and HIV antibody status.

4. To examine the uptake and reactions of gay and bisexual men to 'safer sex' practices (for example the use of condoms).

The main centres of the project are London and South Wales in which a controlled cohort of some 750 men is being studied from 1988 to 1991. Further parallel samples are also being studied in other urban areas to assess regional variations in lifestyle.

The use of diaries and the evaluation of social networking are valuable tools. This can be illustrated by considering the pressure put on men and women who have sex with persons of the same sex in situations where they might be inclined to seek out a sexual experience. The pressure will only be dealt with adequately by empowering them with sufficient life skills to keep their resolve about safer sex and good health in situations where they may meet other people who may not have the same resolve or concern. The diary will show the relevance of situations in which they are likely to seek, or be approached for, a sexual encounter. Analysis should not fall into the trap of implying or assuming that they are any more promiscuous (however defined) than heterosexual people. The most popular meeting places may be: pubs, clubs, bars; discotheques; private parties; gay recreational clubs, youth clubs etc.; public lavatories; saunas and massage parlours; cinemas; public parks or other places known as meeting places for gay people, and also private contact advertisements and phone lines.

Chapter 4

A child with HIV

This chapter will explore the use of the social network approach by considering a case study of a child 'Beth' (aged two) born with HIV and subsequently fostered and adopted by 'Mr and Mrs Rankin'. Before the case study, however, there will be a consideration of some of the key issues pertinent to the care of young children living with HIV infection.

Introduction

The vast majority (80%) of children with HIV have maternally acquired the infection. The mechanisms for infection are:

- intrauterine (cross-placental) transmission
- infection during the birth process (theoretically possible but rare)
- breast feeding. (Breast milk as a route of transmission has been indicated in very few cases worldwide)

The women who have become pregnant and have been found to be HIV positive have either received an unscreened blood transfusion with HIV present or a semen donation for artificial insemination from an HIV seropositive donor, or else have participated in an HIV high risk activity. The latter activities can be defined as:

- injecting drug use with a sharing of equipment (drug 'works')
- participation in unsafe sex as the sexual partner of a seropositive man or woman
- engaging in sex industry work and combining the work with the aforementioned risk activities

In the early years of HIV knowledge (largely based on the situation of black and Hispanic mothers and babies with HIV in America) it was confidently predicted that around 50% of pregnant women with HIV would give birth to a baby who would be infected with HIV and 50% of these babies would go develop AIDS and die within two years. This gloomy scenario has not been noted in the United Kingdom. Dr J Mok,[1] has, for example, noted only low infection rate from HIV positive mothers to children. Children who are born HIV positive appear to be so as the result of carrying maternal antibodies to the virus. Between 75% and 90% of these children appeared to lose maternal viral antibodies between six and 18 months. For this reason the testing of children for

HIV is not considered diagnostically useful until the child is 18 months old. The medical future for children who become clear of HIV antibodies is at present uncertain and they will require periodic testing for HIV and follow-up for some time.

It is important that counselling for HIV pregnant women should take account of these facts. Abortion should not be offered as the appropriate solution especially as there now appears little evidence that the birth process itself is a major co-factor in converting a woman with HIV into one who will develop an AIDS opportunistic infection. Many women with HIV have a strong desire for a family. They may well be socially and financially disadvantaged and as a consequence see little hope for the future. For these women, giving birth may well be the only real affirmation left for them of being of worth as a human sexual being. It should not be assumed that the female drug user's lifsetyle is so disorganised and chaotic as always to render her unfit to be a mother. This may be the position for a minority of women but substitute care should only be considered after a careful social work assessment which takes due cognisance of the human and legal rights of the mother as well as the rights of the child. Other pregnancy related factors formerly associated with drug use should also be treated with caution, in particular, disturbed menstrual periods or erratic sexual activity. (It does not appear that opiate abuse affects fertility as was formerly thought.) Certain clinical co-factors do, however, appear to influence the possibility of maternal transmission of HIV, chief amongst these being:

- the general health of the mother with HIV
- the genetic variability in susceptibility to HIV infection
- the presence of other sexually transmitted disease infections

For a detailed discussion of the spectrum of HIV infection in children, reference should be made to Chapter 3 of *The Implications of AIDS for Children in Care*, published in 1987 by the British Agencies for Adoption and Fostering.

Services for children born with HIV

Hospital services

Children with HIV are usually required to attend a paediatric hospital clinic every three to six months for clinical examination, developmental screening, appropriate tests, immunisations etc. For those children with signs of HIV disease, intravenous infusions of immunoglobulin may be required and therapeutic treatment with drugs such as AZT or Septrin. Attendance at the clinic gives the paediatrician, paramedical and hospital social service staff an important opportunity to give the parents (natural or foster) appropriate support, counselling, information and advice.

Community health services

The role of general practitioners, community nurses and health visitors is invaluable in monitoring the treatment and care of children with HIV. It is considered that as the majority of these children will not show signs of HIV infection they should be integrated as fully as possible into the normal community-based health service system.

Social services

A diagnosis of HIV infection in a child will mean that families will be confronted with all the stigma, isolation, uncertainty and challenges of living with HIV infection. Where parent(s) and child are infected the level of associated problems on a personal and material level are likely to be substantial. It is for this reason that each family will have to be assessed carefully to determine how its coping mechanisms will respond to the problems and issues posed by HIV. In addition to the issues surrounding the physical and emotional well-being of the family, there will be issues, for example, concerning financial resources, the adequacy of housing, the availability of emotional support within and outside the nuclear family. Added to this particular Pandora's box there may be considerations concerning the person's lifestyle that led to the infection of the child in the first place. For all these reasons social care agencies have a key role to play in the support of children and families living with HIV. For this support and care to be given in a way that respects the rights of families and children it is essential that services are provided within a policy framework that preserves these rights.

The principles which can underpin the service provision can be detailed as:

1. The child's needs must have priority when selecting the most suitable service.

2. Agencies should do all they can to help the natural parents to care for their child using all available supports and, if necessary, creating new support systems to meet this goal.

3. Wherever possible, to avoid further stigmatisation and marginalisation of the child with HIV, services should be provided within the normal existing service framework. It is not necessary to create special units for these children.

4. The principle of confidentiality of parent and child is paramount. Where a disclosure of the child's sero-status has to be made it should always be done with the parents' full knowledge and agreement and on the principle of 'who needs to know and why'.

5. Carers (foster parents, day carers (child minders), nursery carers, family centres, play groups, domiciliary supporters) should be given good preparation, training and support in respect of HIV so that they are able to make informed decisions about their willingness to be involved.

6. The stresses involved in caring for a child with HIV will require extra back-up and support.

The ethos in which the care and support are provided is also important. To create this ethos it is vital to remember that any help offered and action taken must be delivered in as caring, compassionate and non-judgemental a manner as possible. The creation of this environment does not, however, diminish the need for a careful assessment of any 'risk' to the child's emotional, physical and intellectual well-being and development. The risk assessment will be multi-factorial and will include lifestyles, environments, and social networks in addition to the well being of the child with HIV. As such, this risk assessment is essentially similar to processes that social workers are already familiar with when determining whether or not the child should remain with his or her natural parents. In the case study to be considered the risk assessment determined that fostering and then adoption was the best course of action.

Fostering a child with HIV

Reference should be made to the Bibliography which outlines source material where more detailed discussion of this subject can be found. The underpinning principle has been well described, however, by the British Association of Social Workers:[2]

> 'Each child will have an individual set of circumstances which should be taken into account when placement is being considered. Just as special health needs are always a factor when deciding on a placement so a child's virus status will have to be taken into account. The process of 'normalisation' should not deny that the virus status confers special needs but rather that those special needs should be assessed and met through established good fostering practice.'

Good practice should come about through a planned programme of preparation and support for foster parents. Such a programme should include:

1. Giving information about HIV:

2. Checking the foster parents' understanding of HIV, Hepatitis B and other relevant infectious diseases:

3. A discussion of routine hygiene measures which (to avoid discrimination) should be implemented on the basis that all children placed with foster parents could be potentially infectious. An infection control procedure should be drawn up by departments, shared with foster parents and implemented through the provision of appropriate information and resources.

4. Establishing contact points in order to avoid foster parents having to battle with bureaucracy to locate the support and information they require.

5. Using the existing group support framework for foster parents. Where this does not exist a framework should urgently be established. Consideration should be given to setting up an additional support group for foster parents/adopters caring for a child with HIV. (Note the use of such a group in the case study to be considered.)

6. Enabling foster parents to 'opt-in' to caring for a child with HIV on the basis of full knowledge of HIV rather than being expected to care for a child with HIV, irrespective. Opting-in will invariably be a family decision once family attitudes to

HIV, sexuality, drug use, confidentiality issues, sickness and mortality concerns have been explored and talked over with key supporters.

7. Fully and appropriately informing all foster parents about the background and (where known) serostatus of the child placed in their care. It is not thought necessary for social workers of other children placed with the foster parent to be routinely informed.

8. Reviewing and monitoring all placements by the social work agency in a way that is supportive and not intimidating for the foster family.

Adopting a child with HIV

Initially the 'state of the art' of caring for children with HIV rarely considered adoption as a realistic possibility. The special health needs of these children were seen as requiring some specialist, often segregated resource. It was therefore incredibly uplifting for the researcher to meet (in the case study that follows) a child like 'Beth' and adopters like the 'Rankins' where Beth's needs for permanency in her primary relationships were being met in a secure and emotionally happy environment despite the ever present fears of a possible reduced life expectancy. Some of the issues for adopters of children with HIV are, therefore, seen as follows:

1. The uncertainty of knowing whether a child will, (if they become free of antibodies to the virus) still progress to HIV chronic infection and possibly AIDS.

2. If the child survives, what kind of life can it expect given the probable sexual limits on relationships and childbearing imposed by HIV.

3. Helping a child understand the reality of his or her adopted status is a challenge in itself without the additional complications of having to assimilate some knowledge and comprehension of their antibody status. The potential emotional vulnerability of coming to terms with adoption could, for a child, be doubly intensified by having to take on board the implications of HIV. A child with HIV should be told sensitively about HIV when they are well and before they reach adolescence. Children are often very capable of assimilating this knowledge and adults should not assume the child will react as they would react.

4. What are the prospects for adopters adopting another child if they have already adopted a child with HIV infection?

5. What effect will the adoption of an HIV positive child have on the family and their social network? Will the child and the family be ostracised by other family members, friends, neighbours, colleagues at work?

6. How will issues around confidentiality be handled within the family? With the babysitter? With the local school?

For these reasons, amongst others, counselling at the initial stages of the adoption process coupled with information and support will be just as crucial as the need for appropriate follow up support.

Beth - an adopted child

Kirsty and Mike Rankin have been married for fifteen years. They are both 35 years old. Fairly early on in their marriage they discovered that they would not be able to have a child of their own. Kirsty and Mike then applied to their local authority for registration as foster-parents but were turned down as being too young and not having enough experience. The time taken to reach the decision was more annoying for them than the decision itself but they re-applied seven years later and this time their application was accepted and they were approved very quickly. Since then they have had many short-stay foster children and have an expertise recognised by their local department for taking hard-to-place young children.

Kirsty and Mike live in a rural area characterised by local coal mining. They are about ten miles from a major city. Their family network contacts are, in the main, fairly close by or within easy driving distance. Mike works as a television repair operative. The family live in a three-bedroom modern terrace house having moved there recently partly because of the fears that Beth's natural mother might try to trace them as she had threatened to do. Currently, apart from the family dog Bonnie 'a stray that adopted us five years ago' the Rankins are also foster parents to five-year-old twins. These twins presented severe behaviour problems when living with their family in overcrowded accommodation. When first placed with the Rankins the twins were very uncontrolled, shouting, running about, throwing things, kicking walls, screaming and head banging. Although the twins' behaviour has somewhat moderated they still present problems in management. 'Walk to calm foster children down' features in the week's diary kept for the researcher by Kirsty and Mike (see *Figure 15*). The tantrums thrown by the twins is a factor to be considered when Beth is in their close proximity as she could easily be hurt.

Beth's natural mother Louise is an injecting drug user who has had three children adopted and a subsequent abortion. This is despite the fact that during most of this period she had been HIV positive as a result of needle sharing. Last heard about, Louise had been an inmate in a woman's prison and had become drug free as a result. It is unlikely, given what is known about Louise, that she will not drift back into the drug using scene. Louise had regular social work counselling throughout this period in respect of:

(a) Her drug use.

(b) The need to place Beth with foster parents.

(c) The organisation for any contact and access she could have with Beth.

(d) The adoption process.

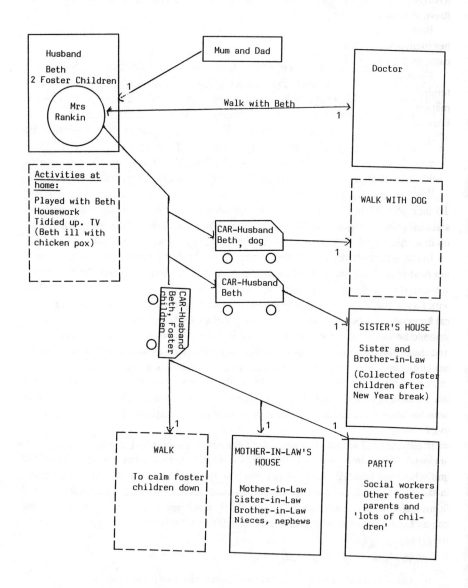

Fig. 15 - A week in Mrs Rankin's life with Beth

Louise's contact with her daughter became erratic and unpredictable. There was always a fear for the Rankins that she might turn up and try to remove Beth, hence their recent move of house.

Beth was placed with Kirsty and Mike when she was four weeks old. They describe her then as a '2 lb 6 oz baby with a great personality' who quickly put on weight and became an appealing and very manageable baby.

From the outset Kirsty and Mike were aware of Beth's seropositivity, having attended a foster parent group which had enabled them to decide, on the basis of information given, that they would be prepared to take a baby with HIV. They felt that they knew the score 'warts and all'. As Kirsty put it:

'We decided we would deal with the child first - a small girl who needed love and attention the same as any other child - and deal with the distress of her becoming ill if and when that happened. We know we'll have the warnings, and we know we'll get the back up.'

To their surprise, Kirsty and Mike also developed a degree of sympathy and understanding for Louise and other drug users, whom they describe as 'young people caught up in something so difficult to stop'.

In the initial days Beth required a sustained level of hospital follow-up to monitor her health, in particular to assess whether she would remain asymptomatic or whether she would develop any of the physiological and neurological complications associated with HIV infection. Because Beth was in many ways at the forefront of emerging medical knowledge about HIV infection in children a strong bond of support and trust developed between the hospital paediatrician and the Rankins. The regular hospital visits and the blood tests have, however, been a strain for Beth. Kirsty has had to draw on all her strengths of consoling to help the little girl cope with the associated trauma of these visits (injections, investigations etc). No matter how sensitive the system, the health trauma will always be there as Beth moves into her school years. The effects should not be underestimated and ways to minimise any stress will always need to be sought out and evaluated. Currently three-monthly tests and examinations involve checking development as well as taking nose and throat swabs and blood tests. Major hospital examinations take place on a six-monthly basis for Beth. The little girl has continued to flourish and appears to be developing normally. She has lost antibodies to the virus and on her last two tests has remained seronegative. During the period in which the researcher was in contact with the Rankins and Beth she developed chicken pox (see *Figure 15*) and in consequence the next test is awaited with a degree of anxiety in case the infection has triggered any HIV associated reaction. The primary medical care for Beth has now been transferred to the community based medical services with the general practitioner and health visitor taking on key roles. The chicken pox infection in itself necessitated special medication for Beth. The Rankins are used to the need for special consideration over what would be routine treatments, such as antibiotics and immunisations because of the very nature and unpredictability of HIV infection. Initially, live vaccines were not used but now it is felt that measles and mumps pose a greater danger. Hence normal vaccinations processes are followed except for the use of inactivated polio vaccinations.

Despite the adoption process, Kirsty and Mike recognised that, because of HIV, in many ways their bonding with Beth might be more profound and special than with the other children who had been placed with them on a short term basis. For this reason, in 1987, they decided to seek to adopt Beth. This adoption was completed in the middle of 1988, nearly a year and a half after Beth was first placed with them. The Rankins have already done some preparatory thinking about when and how to tell Beth about the adoption, supplementing this with information prepared in a child's book on adoption and information given in letter form by Louise. At present they see it as a priority to take it a step at a time.

Network analysis

The diary kept by Kirsty and Mike for the researcher (see *Figure 15*) clearly indicates the places and activities that are significant in their daily living with Beth, taking account of the care and support needs for Beth and the family. Consideration of networking shows three key focal areas:

1. Extended family support.
2. Health support systems.
3. Social service support systems.

1. Extended family support system

Both Kirsty and Mike have extensive family networks. These are shown in *Figures 16* and *17*. In the main, family live close by or within easy driving distance. The significance and benefit of the networks to Kirsty and Mike can also be assessed using the 'model relationship qualities' developed by Philip Seed.[3]

(i) Communication and access

Do their relationships increase Kirsty and Mike's opportunity to communicate and is this communication aided by accessibility (distance, transport)? Is access gained to other people through shared activities?

(ii) Instrumental qualities

Do their relationships help Kirsty and Mike in practical ways? Are they enabled to do the things they would not otherwise be able to do because of increased practical supports?

(iii) Sentiment qualities

What sort of feelings do Kirsty and Mike have for key people in the social network and how has this influenced whether they have shared the knowledge of their daughter's

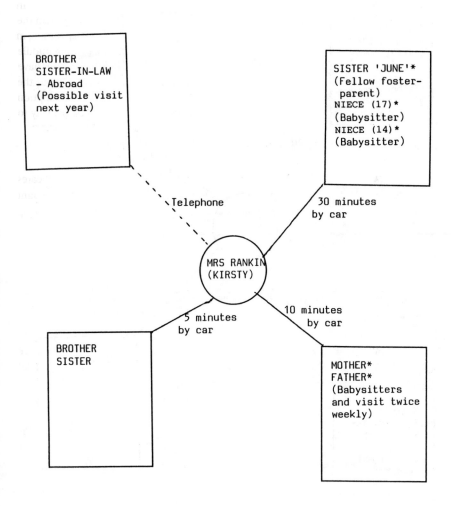

BROTHER
SISTER-IN-LAW
- Abroad
(Possible visit
next year)

SISTER 'JUNE'*
(Fellow foster-
   parent)
NIECE (17)*
(Babysitter)
NIECE (14)*
(Babysitter)

Telephone

30 minutes
by car

MRS RANKIN
(KIRSTY)

5 minutes
by car

10 minutes
by car

BROTHER
SISTER

MOTHER*
FATHER*
(Babysitters
and visit twice
weekly)

* indicates these people (only) know of Beth's HIV status.

Fig. 16 - Extended family network of Mrs Rankin (Kirsty)

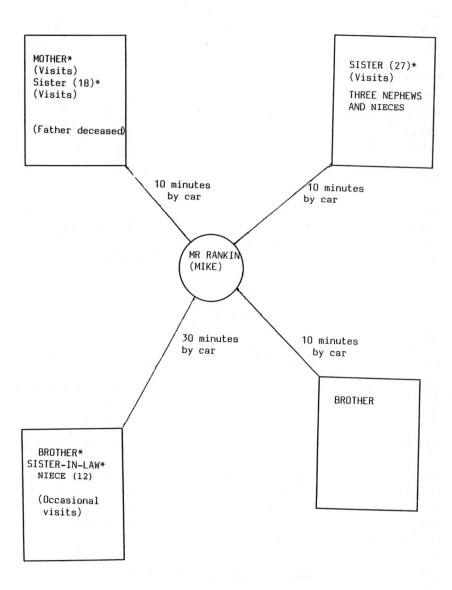

MOTHER*
(Visits)
Sister (18)*
(Visits)

(Father deceased)

SISTER (27)*
(Visits)

THREE NEPHEWS
AND NIECES

10 minutes
by car

10 minutes
by car

MR RANKIN
(MIKE)

30 minutes
by car

10 minutes
by car

BROTHER

BROTHER*
SISTER-IN-LAW*
NIECE (12)

(Occasional
visits)

* indicates these people (only) know of Beth's HIV status.

Fig. 17 - Extended family network of Mr Rankin (Mike)

seropositivity or not? Feelings expressed may be around admiration, hostility, sociability, reliability. In what ways does the expression of these feelings help Kirsty and Mike?

(iv) Reciprocal qualities

Are Kirsty and Mike able to reciprocate help to 'key others' in the network practically or by facilitation of communication and feelings?

This analysis can be extended to include an analysis of Kirsty and Mike's relationships with friends and officials (health, social work, education, others). A value in using this analysis is that it not only identifies gaps in support but also highlights any possible areas of duplication.

Kirsty and Mike have moved recently because of their anxiety that Louise would trace them and try and remove Beth. The move was within a ten mile radius and they have a car. There is no evidence that there is a significant loss or benefit from the move to the new living situation. There is some slight diminution of support from neighbours (there are new neighbours whom they do not know yet) but the move has not removed them significantly from supports within the family and health and social work support systems.

The 17-year-old niece is taking her driving test which, if she passes, will improve her accessibility and potential to babysit. Both nieces have no problem maintaining the necessary confidentiality about Beth. Kirsty and Mike hope to visit their relatives abroad and are contemplating sharing the news about Beth prior to that visit. They speak positively of this brother and they have more contact with him than with the local brother and sister where there is relatively less support, and no sharing of the child's serostatus. The brother and his family are described as 'not very social people' despite the close accessibility.

Kirsty's sister June (who is also a foster parent) plays a crucial role in providing support. Although living 30 minutes away contact is regular by car, with the sister and niece providing babysitting services and also allowing their house to be used as a pick up and drop point for the five-year-old twins (Kirsty and Mike's foster children). They are collected by the twin's social worker before onward transportation to their own family. 'The instrumental qualities' analysis shows benefits for Kirsty and Mike in this relationship and there is a mutuality of peer-support through Kirsty's own support of June's foster placements. Kirsty and her sister attend the local authority special support group for foster parents prepared to take an HIV child and June is awaiting the opportunity to foster an HIV baby. The common experience of caring for an HIV baby means that Kirsty, June and June's daughter are fully conversant with the necessary health and hygiene procedures that require to be implemented. Babysitting support is important because it enables Mike and Kirsty to have a much needed break from Beth and the twins and relax.

The diary (*Figure 15*) also shows Kirsty and June attending a New Year party for foster parents run by the local authority attended by 'social workers, other foster parents and lots of children'.

Mike describes his family as seeing each other mostly around Christmas, New Year and birthday. The social interaction is far less frequent and intense than Kirsty's. The diary which was completed at the New Year shows the importance of Mike's mother's house as a central point for family gathering. The impression the researcher gained was that the information given to the family about Beth was less detailed. One brother was not told about Beth and HIV because it was considered that his girlfriend was 'not very stable' and could react badly or breach confidentiality. It was not felt that the time was right to share any information with the 12-year-old niece.

Sharing Information

Confidentiality and sharing of information about a child's HIV status are clearly areas that have to be handled with caution and sensitivity. For Kirsty and Mike the need carefully to weigh up whom to tell about Beth and the consideration of other children within the family are both issues which have been shared with their social worker. The guidelines for 'telling' prepared by the local authority have been helpfully explicit on these points:

(i) The only people who must be told are the General Practitioner, the health visitor and other doctors treating the child.

(ii) Do not share the information with anyone else without first discussing it with your social worker. The natural parent's right to be consulted must be respected. (Once adoption has been formalised this right ceases in law.)

(iii) Sharing of information is only necessary where there are special medical considerations or where the actual care of the child is transferred to someone else either frequently or for long periods of time.

(iv) Foster parents are the best judge of whether their own children need to know. It is sensible, however, to make sure that everyone in the family knows about HIV and the need for appropriate hygiene.

(v) The burden of secrecy is hard to carry alone. When it is necessary to share information about the child's seropositivity with a relative, friend, babysitter, etc, foster parents should take time to consider this need with the social worker.

The advice of the British National Fostercare Association is also very useful:

'If temporary carers and professionals are educated about the need for good hygiene in respect of all children, the need to pass information about any child's specific infection is reduced considerably.'[4]

Injudicious sharing of information could result in a child being unfairly excluded from playgroups and nursery provisions. Friends may not visit and the family may feel rejected because of prejudice and lack of understanding about HIV infection. The question therefore needs to be reiterated: 'who needs to know and why?'

After careful consideration, Kirsty and Mike decided to tell the head teacher of the local school to which Beth will go when she is five. This head teacher has already had contact with the family because of the twins' attendance and Kirsty and Mike felt comfortable and confident about how the teacher would handle the information. Reassuringly, their confidence was not misplaced! This sharing of information was decided upon despite the Education Department's policy that schools do not need to be informed when a child has HIV, staff having been given guidance about standards of hygiene for all children to prevent spread of infections including HIV.

2. Health network

For Beth the health network is as follows:

- city based hospital - three to six monthly visit
- General Practitioner - as necessary
- health visitor - monthly
- dentist - (future consideration)

The links between the hospital paediatrician and the General Practitioner were very important when Beth developed chicken pox. Advice was sought and special medication subsequently prescribed. The Rankins are very happy with the contact they have received from the consultant paediatrician and their own doctor. The researcher asked them to rate the services they had received from health and social workers on the basis of a standardised system of scoring, identifying degrees of satisfaction or dissatisfaction with services received:

Score Key Phrases

1 Very satisfied (excellent)

2 Fairly satisfied (good)

3 Neither satisfied or dissatisfied (acceptable but not good)

4 Rather dissatisfied (not good enough)

5 Very dissatisfied (deplorable)

Both the consultant paediatrician and the General Practitioner scored 1. Kirsty and Mike's criteria for this rating were:

- time spent with us
- ability to share information in a way that we understood
- general information and advice
- warmth of personality and 'relatability'
- how the doctor handled Beth ('confidence breeds confidence')

The Rankins have had two health visitors. Whereas health visitor B (current) rated 1, health visitor A only rated 3. Health visitor 'A' was described as being 'stand-offish' 'needing to put on aprons and gloves when handling the child, and disinfecting the scales'. Her competence was not in question, but her attitudes seemed to the Rankins to reinforce fear and anxiety about HIV. Health visitor B (rating 1), in contrast, is described as someone who is 'relaxed', 'a person one could have a right old chat with'. 'She gives useful information'. In contrast to the 'gloved up' approach of health visitor 'A' the current health visitor puts her fingers in Beth's mouth and treats her like any other child. Kirsty recognised her own inexperience when Beth came to her as a foster child. She was limited in her experience of babies and lived 'by the rules'. She felt she could have received more back up support than she received, especially over 'feeds'. Now her anxiety level is considerably abated and she is approaching the prospect of potty training with equanimity and support from health visitor B.

Kirsty and Mike see that they will soon need to seek advice and think through the need (or otherwise) to inform their dentist about Beth. Given the fact that dental services should be provided on the basis of good health and infection control procedures, it should not be necessary to pass information on about Beth. However, as discussed, dental care of children with HIV is in its relative infancy and it may well be in Beth's interest for the same supportive links to be established between paediatrician and dentist as exist between paediatrician and GP. Some hospitals provide their own dental services for children with HIV.

3. Social service networks

The level and nature of the support to foster parent and adopters of children with HIV given by social services departments seems the vital component to the success of the placement. Many potentially difficult issues surround the placement. Some of these can be identified (in general) as:

(i) Uncertainty over the child's health career.

(ii) Will the child return to his or her natural home and, if so, when and to what situation?

(iii) What access will the natural parents have and how will the foster family cope, especially if there is a risk that the turbulent family background and drug lifestyle will transfer to the foster family situation.

(iv) How to deal with confidentiality issues.

(v) The need for continued advice and information about HIV and related matters, e.g. the handling of the child's developing sexuality.

(vi) Relating to a range of professionals who may have differing levels of HIV knowledge and abilities in dealing with HIV and AIDS.

The support, counselling and back up that foster parents and adopters receive both in a one-to-one and group setting are crucial. Some local authorities have identified key organisational issues which need to be addressed:

(i) Establishing an effective network between professionals so that consistent information is exchanged and common treatment goals are identified where possible.

(ii) Updating information and advice about the developing HIV knowledge base and ensuring that this is communicated to, and assimilated by, key social service staff.

(iii) Dealing with uncertainty can be as stressful for staff as it is for carers. Staff may feel de-skilled, anxious, very tired for example. It is essential, therefore, that supervision, support, and time off (where appropriate) are legitimised by the caring organisation. Unless this is done staff morale will sink and there will be a distinct risk of staff 'burn-out'.

(iv) The institutional tension between specialist and field/residential social workers needs to be acknowledged and managed so that it does not impede the services given.

Kirsty and Mike are in a good position to evaluate the services they have received from their local social services department. Their network shows a high-level interface with social workers (specialist, liaison, managerial):

- Beth's social worker visits as and when required
- liaison social worker visits at least monthly
- twins' social worker visits at least monthly
- AIDS Advisor visits at least quarterly

There is also a special group for foster parents and adopters of children with HIV. The group was set up in the Autumn of 1987 and meets monthly. It is facilitated by a senior social worker, AIDS advisor and family placement staff. The aims of the group are broadly:

1. To offer support, information and advice to substitute carers of a child with HIV.

2. To allow carers to compare similarities in coping strategies.

3. To allow carers to expand their coping strategies.

4. To allow the expression of 'bottled-up' feelings in a safe environment.

5. To allow ventilation of feelings about existing services.

Crèche facilities are available. Some weeks the group meets purely for mutual support and sharing experiences: at other times the paediatrician will give regular updates on HIV knowledge and services. The group has also been featured in the media and met a well known personality with HIV. The latter proved an exhilarating experience for Kirsty and Mike. They described the powerful and supportive impact the group session had for them in meeting an adult with HIV who was asymptomatic and living a positively healthy life. It gave them great encouragement in perceiving a rosier future for their little daughter than they had initially imagined. Finally, they attend a local foster parent support group which meets monthly.

Using the same 'degree of satisfaction' score described earlier, Kirsty and Mike rated their liaison social worker 1 on the basis that the social worker was:

- a person they felt 'relaxed' with
- somebody prepared to admit that he did not know all the answers but would find out the information they needed
- someone who played with Beth and allowed her to 'drool all over his briefcase'

They admitted to having had negative experiences with social workers in the past, particularly those who had been keen to impress them with their qualifications and who gave them the impression of having 'done it all'. Kirsty put it in a nutshell when she told the researcher:

'they might have been to University but we have been through the University of Life'.

An analysis of the week in the life of Kirsty, Mike and Beth taken at New Year showed the importance played by the family, health and social service networks. Kirsty and Mike are a couple very dedicated to their role as foster parents. They support each other, the family supports them and the social work and health support system act as integral back up systems. The week was, in a sense, atypical, in that it was a New Year week when Mike was home on holiday. Therefore, he features more highly in journeying with his wife than he would in a normal week. The car is very important to the family as it enables them to link with the various contact points in the networks and also gave them the ability to go for a walk to a local beauty spot when the twins had been particularly fractious and again when their dog needed a walk.

Network analysis should also consider the role of animals. Bonnie (a very affectionate creature as the researcher was quick to discover!) acts not only as a household pet but also as a valuable asset in helping Beth's development and ability to walk. Bonnie also played an important role in helping the twins to settle down and in defusing their aggression. The role of animals in children's homes, foster placements and in the ordinary family home should never be underestimated. The Rankin's diary shows a normal busy household dividing its weekly activities between those commonly associated with household life and those activities specifically associated with Beth's serostatus and ongoing follow-up.

Conclusion

In America, special children's homes have been established to care for toddlers and young children with HIV. These homes are called 'Grandma homes' because the grandmother is seen as a traditional bedrock of the family. They are a symbol of the unqualified love, understanding, strength and security so desperately needed in AIDS care. For the researcher, however, the study of Beth and her family shows most powerfully that this love, strength and security are achievable in a household in a community and in a way that did not stigmatise or discriminate. As such the future for Beth and children like her must be filled with qualified yet realistic hope.

Caring for children like Beth will remain a challenge for natural families, substitute carers and involved professionals. Policies will need to be evolved by organisations that are flexible enough to deal with new HIV issues as and when they arise but that are not so all encompassing as to lead to the creation of overdependency on the system. Key to success in the caring task is the partnership which should exist between the various elements of the support network and the family of the child with HIV.

Points for discussion

1. What issues are most important for (a) fostering and (b) adopting a child with HIV infection?

2. Assess the strengths and weaknesses of Kirsty and Mike as if you were assessing them as adoptive parents for Beth.

3. How would you advise Kirsty and Mike regarding their fear that Louise, Beth's natural mother, might 'turn up'.

4. Consider the question of whom to tell about the HIV status of a adopted child. Examine this in relation to the information given in *Figures 16* and *17*.

5. Discuss the Rankins' views of the health and social service workers in their health and social service networks. How could these services be improved?

6. What part do animals play in Beth's social network?

7. What constraints will Beth's HIV uncertainty place on Beth's future development?

8. What constraints will Beth's HIV uncertainty place on the Rankin's family life in the future?

9. What particular social work skills are most important in working with this family?

10. How should services be developed in ways that do not undermine the parents of a child with HIV?

References

1. Mok, J. K., et. al. (1987), 'Infants Born To Mothers Seropositive for HIV'. *The Lancet*, 1987, 1164-8
2. BASW. *HIV-AIDS. A Social Work Perspective.*
3. Seed, P. (1989), *Network Analysis in Social Work*, London: Jessica Kingsley Publishers.
4. (1981), *AIDS and HIV. Information for Foster Parents*, National Foster Care Association publications.

Chapter 5

Support for relatives and partners of people living with HIV and AIDS

This chapter will explore the situation of lovers, partners and families of people with HIV and AIDS and describe the work of a support group set up for them in one British city.

By its very nature HIV is a condition which has affected primarily those who are young, sexually active and independent. Some of these people will live with or near families (c.f. Ryan, *Chapter 3*). Others will have grown away from the family and will now be faced with difficult decisions over informing relatives about the illness, their sexual orientation or drug use and their possible mortality. Sharing the knowledge of HIV infection with partners will also present a major challenge not only in the telling but also, by its implications, to the stability of the relationship. In turn, partners and family members may be left feeling numb and helpless as a result of these revelations. Invariably, they will go through the same feelings as the person diagnosed with HIV. A range of feelings and fears (some irrational) will have to be faced up to. These include:

1. Fear of being infected with the virus now or in the future.

2. Guilt at being the possible infector.

3. Isolation and feeling of stigma caused by the perceived (real or imaginary) reaction of other friends, neighbours, family members, etc.

4. Isolation from the person with HIV. (Partners and families may experience a feeling of premature loss of intimacy through difficulties in relating to a person sexually or even by touch, hug, kiss and so forth.)

5. Isolation at the prospect of separation from the loved one by either hospitalisation or death.

6. Anger and grief because of such an illness in a young person.

7. Anger at the person or the situation believed to be the cause of infection.

8. Feelings of self recrimination, devastation, or being overwhelmed by the unknown and unpredictable nature of the virus and its disease progression.

9. Feeling a need to take over and care totally for the person with HIV.

10. Guilt because of one's partner's or relatives' sexual orientation or drug using life style.

11. For the haemophiliac and his family there will be many feelings associated with the genetic and medical transmission of the virus as well as the feelings of 'disease' caused by being HIV positive.

Many of these feelings (especially the stigma) will be exacerbated if the person with HIV begins to develop symptoms of chronic HIV infection and AIDS, particularly those symptoms associated with body image: loss of body weight, looks (Kaposi's lesions) - tumours, body rashes, loss of hair, etc.

For the person with HIV, their partner and family, it may well be very difficult to deal with these feelings. Other terminal illnesses, for example, may be used to find a more socially acceptable and less stigmatising diagnosis with which to inform others. In short, families or partnerships will often turn inwards so that the experience for them becomes private, trapped, unexpressed, avoided and the emotional sequelae never really worked through.

The dependency created by HIV and AIDS in its more florid stages is often compounded by a health and social service system that in itself is not only destructive of independence but also often forces the person living with HIV and AIDS and their family further and further into a dependent role. 'Experts' (doctors, psychologists, social workers, AIDS counsellors,) tend to take over to the point that their ministration can actually run the risk of becoming health debilitating and death accelerating. It is to fight this image of HIV dependence that groups like 'Positively Healthy' have recently been set up, opening up as they have a range of options both in terms of health and life style not totally dependent on drugs like AZT (with its known toxicity risks as well as its benefits). To counteract this unmitigating sense of dependency and loss of control over one's own destiny, groups are now being set up to address the needs of people with HIV and the needs of their carers and key members of their social and family networks. In this way it is hoped that care for people living with HIV and AIDS can be integrated with, rather than run parallel to, support services for their relatives, lovers and partners. For this, however, to be achieved with any degree of effectiveness, it is argued that a three way relationship has to be established on the basis of the model shown in *Figure 18*.

The adoption of this model should achieve the promotion of personal independence, greater flexibility of services, more enlightened systems of caring, aggressive health promotion and, above all, more choice for the consumer. While social policies and social services remain locked into the notion of HIV pathology, many of the intrinsic rights of people living with HIV and AIDS will run the risk of being substantially eroded - in particular, the right to participate in their own health care and the rights associated with confidentiality. In some cases, the right of a service may be denied as, for example, there is some evidence that General Practitioners may be becoming increasingly reluctant to have drug users or homosexual men on their lists. Even when a service can be provided it has been noted that people with, or at risk of, HIV infection may be reluctant to take up these services because of real or perceived censorious and homophobic attitudes of the service providers. Families, partners and relatives experience and share many of the

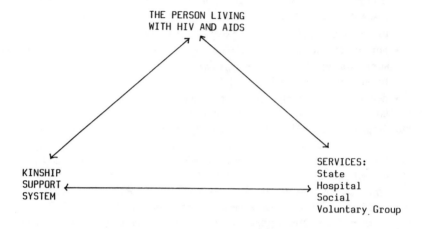

Fig. 18 - Model of a three-way support relationship

associated feelings, particularly the isolation, with their loved one with HIV and often
deal with the same dependency creating services. Groups have, therefore, been set up
to ensure that relatives and partners may find comfort, new knowledge and independence. The researcher was able to visit one such group BRIDGE (not its real name).
This is a support group for partners, families and close friends of people with HIV or
AIDS.

'BRIDGE' grew out of the shared experiences of two hospital senior social workers
with people with HIV in separate hospitals where gay men and drug users were seen
regularly for HIV pre-test counselling, testing, post- test follow up and treatment. The
counselling the social workers provided brought them regularly in touch with the
families of the people with HIV and it was noted that many common factors emerged
from this counselling, in particular:

- the stress caused by the HIV diagnosis
- the need for more knowledge and information
- the reactions and fears of relatives and partners (particularly of the HIV unknown
  and isolation)

- confidentiality and 'who needs to know?' within the family. (e.g. how do you share the information with children?)
- how to handle the reaction of other people not within the nuclear or extended family
- how to build back their own social networking. (Some relatives, for example, had stopped going to the pub, feeling it could be hurtful for the person with HIV who through illness or self imposed isolation wished to remain at home.)
- dealing with bureaucracies (Health, Benefits services and Social Services in particular)
- feelings about the media. (During 1987 when families were coming to terms with the reality of HIV within the family, they were exposed to repeated 'assaults' about HIV and AIDS in the media, much of which gave conflicting advice and much of which, especially in the papers, was prejudiced and downright hurtful to the families.)The social workers realised that these feelings could be dealt with through 'old fashioned one-to-one casework' but it quickly became apparent that there was another common request being made by these relatives. It could be summed up thus: 'they (the people with HIV) have got *Body Positive*. It is a pity there is nothing similar for us'. It was out of this concern that BRIDGE evolved.

The first need was to set up some ground rules for the group and this was done by focussing on some of the key issues and needs which, when identified, were drawn together in an introductory pamphlet. The key issues were:

1. Confidentiality

When setting up the group there was a fear that, in sharing information, the relative/carer might inadvertantly identify the person with HIV for whom they cared. The social workers (who became the group leaders/facilitators) felt that members should only introduce themselves by their Christian names. Where possible, it was felt that the carer should inform the person with HIV that they were attending the group but that they should not talk about the group discussions. The importance of the confidential nature of the group discussions was felt to be of paramount importance.

2. Funding

BRIDGE required a small budget to cover running costs. These costs were seen to be carer's travelling expenses, refreshments and the purchase and hire of educational material. These running costs were subsequently met by a local AIDS charity.

3. Premises/Membership

The premises identified were city centre based although the group itself was not confined to people from the immediate city area but was open to relatives and carers from the surrounding rural areas. The only common factor was the attendance of the person with HIV at some time at the city centre hospitals.

4. Transport

It was recognised that getting to the group was likely to be financially demanding on some members, especially those from the rural areas and those on low incomes. Where hardship was likely to be experienced, transport costs would be considered. (There was not an open ended offer of payment of costs to all members, recognising that this could be insulting and create dependence.)

5. Babysitters

Carers with young families might be put off attending the meetings because they could not afford the cost of a babysitter. If such a situation arose then these costs would also be considered as part of the group's running costs.

For BRIDGE to run successfully and achieve its aims, several key needs were identified, these were:

1. Speakers

For the group to be usefully supportive and meet the need for facts about a disease where knowledge and information is developing daily, speakers with a specialist knowledge should be invited to some of the meetings. These speakers could be health, social work and media related. Speakers whose concern was service delivery should be invited where possible.

2. Pamphlets

To assist with the knowledge and information giving, it was felt that each member of BRIDGE should be given an information pack at the first meeting. The pack would contain a range of leaflets about HIV and AIDS, Harm Reduction, Safer Sex and information about other local groups, clinics and related resources. This provision grew not only out of a need to maximise HIV information but also out of an emphathic recognition that people can feel stigmatised by picking up HIV leaflets on public display.

3. Alleviating stress

The group leaders recognised the need to involve the group members in relaxation and other stress reduction techniques. This recognition grew out of an awareness that caring for someone with HIV or AIDS can lead to a high level of stress for the carer. Stress may be due to:

- fear of the person with HIV developing AIDS and dying

- fear of catching the virus
- anxiety engendered by maintaining confidentiality
- stigma
- possible lifestyle changes

Some of the stress and anxiety may also result from not having accurate information or not knowing about appropriate resources. Furthermore, the knowledge that other people face stress and having the opportunity to share this stress alongside any other problems became, in many ways, the *raison d'être* for BRIDGE and the cornerstone of its continued functioning.

BRIDGE has now run for two ten-week sessions both of which have facilitated the evolution of the ten-week session programme. This has now been adopted for future meetings. The following is a brief description of the programme:

Session 1: **Getting To Know You**

An opportunity for carers to meet and get to know one another, share the ground rules for the group and discuss the structure of the rest of the programme. The information pack will also be distributed.

Session 2: **Information about local HIV groups, clinics, services**

An opportunity to discuss local services and relevant resources and explain their functions. This discussion will use the material already distributed in the fact packs.

Session 3: **Medical input**

An invited speaker will explain HIV and AIDS in layman's terms. The speaker will also respond to any questions, issues and areas of confusion.

Session 4: **Open meeting**

This meeting is an opportunity to review group progress so far, spend time on any issues that have arisen and reflect on the group's future.

Session 5: **Media coverage**

A discussion of how HIV and AIDS has been put across by the media, in particular: newspaper headlines, television campaigns, television plays, advertising and educational videos. This session should help not only to give members a chance to explore their feelings in relation to the media but also dispel myths about the virus.

Session 6: **Exploring attitudes of others**

Continuing from Session 5 the group will examine the stresses and comforts they have felt from the attitudes of others, family, friends, neighbours, work colleagues and professionals. During this session a variety of techniques will be used including group exercises and role plays.

Session 7: Exploring personal attitudes

Continuing from Session 6 the group aims to look at the carer's individual prejudices, stresses and strengths in relation to HIV and AIDS. A similar range of techniques to Session 6 is used.

Session 8: Principal officer (HIV and AIDS)

The Principal Officer from the local social services department is invited to hear the group's views on service provision and perceived gaps in services. The importance of the consumer's view in influencing planning and service delivery is thereby recognised.

Session 9: Open meeting

This meeting provides an opportunity to spend time on the issues which have arisen in the previous four sessions.

Session 10: General review

The BRIDGE group looks at the work undertaken through the whole programme and evaluates the strengths and weaknesses in what it has attempted to achieve.

Each Session usually ends with group time spent in developing relaxation through the use of tapes, music and gentle exercises.

The researcher's interest in the group was known and shared with group members who kindly invited him to one of their open meetings. The researcher was keen to seek their views on;

1. The impact of HIV on family functioning.
2. The impact of HIV on social functioning.
3. Why members felt they had come to the group.
4. Whether there had been any significant changes for the carer or the person cared for as a result of their attendance at the group.

Family functioning

One group member described the difficulties caused by their relative with HIV taking to their bed (despite being asymptomatic) and isolating themselves for a while from the rest of the family. Another spoke about the stresses and anxieties caused to all of them by living with uncertainty. The fear of death was ever present and one 14-year-old boy had had to be referred to a psychologist because of the effect anxiety and stress were having on his home and school life. Whom to tell, and how to involve the person with HIV in sanctioning this knowledge, were key issues. Mothers, 'in-laws', and a grandparent had also not been told for a variety of reasons (see also *Chapter 4* and the description of the Rankin family). Communicating the information (or not) to younger members of the family was a matter of concern. Concern that confidentiality would be kept within the family was also discussed - especially as younger members might find it difficult to 'keep the family secret'. Not talking about HIV, denial and sweeping it under the carpet were also vividly described. All these issues added pressures on the family and influenced how well it functioned. A gay man also described the effect on his home life and on sexual relations through living with a partner who had HIV. HIV was just as much a stress on the partnership as it was for those living in family situations. For the latter, however, it was clear that HIV had probed the very basic fabric of family functioning. Those families who had had difficulties in relationship and communication before the advent of HIV in their lives had found that the added stresses had almost been unbearable and had threatened family stability. Those families in which there was a good 'fit' between members had developed a range of coping skills into which HIV had to some extent been assimilated, although it had been a tremendous challenge.

Social functioning

It was readily apparent to the researcher that social functioning of group members had in a large measure been affected by HIV through the feared reactions of others. In particular:

- the person with HIV had cut themselves off from social contact.
- the person with HIV had started going to the pub more often saying, 'I might as well cram as much in as I can before I die.'
- networking became dominated by the need to attend hospitals, clinics, GPs, etc.
- the effect of physical/mental symptoms on social networking, in particular, 'not feeling well', tiredness, mood swings.
- not wishing to go out socially in case anyone asks awkward questions unless there is a prepared 'socially acceptable response'.
- a fear that 'everyone else knew' was also given as a reason for reducing socialising.

Coming to the group

It was clear to the researcher when he met the group that the members thrived on the opportunity to meet and share experiences. The commonality of the experience of living with the virus in their relationships ensured a sharing of feelings and ideas. This was very therapeutic once a safe and accepting environment had been created by the group facilitators whose role was evident and crucial.

Changes as a result of coming to the group

Group members described these as:

- feeling supported
- being more informed about HIV and local services
- being able to relate better to their relative and partner through an understanding of what they were going through
- being able to stand back and allow decisions to be made by the person with HIV without feeling that they themselves had to come up with a solution
- realising that much about HIV was to do with what was in the mind rather than in fact
- being able to take the media coverage of HIV and AIDS with a pinch of salt and not feeling stigmatised themselves
- being able to express feelings (love, anger, emotional hurts) which had formerly been 'bottled up' for fear of distressing the person with HIV
- feeling less stressed and learning how to relax
- feeling less trapped by HIV and a perceived need to stay at home with the person with the virus
- establishing new friendships with other group members

It was noticeable to the researcher that the group members were also able to share with each other 'negative' (angry) feelings about their relative's or partner's attitudes and response to HIV without feeling guilty. They also felt easier talking about death-related issues where necessary. Although the emphasis of the group life was very much about positive approaches to living with HIV this was not at the expense of allowing purposeful expression of difficult feelings.

Comment

Addressing the World AIDS Summit of Ministers of Health, January 1988, Dr David Miller stated:

'It is vital also to consider the role of 'significant others' in the care of people with AIDS. Carers and loved ones are our main community helpers. Yet good counselling necessitates that they, too, be informed and educated and supported through the post diagnostic period...'[1]

Groups like 'Positive Partners', the Terrence Higgins Trust Family Support Group, and others provide places where members can, in an intimate setting, put aside differences and deal with problems common to them all as a result of HIV infection. To do this requires some role adjustment as carers become, in a sense, cared for themselves. Once a creative supportive environment was achieved, strengths and abilities were developed. Fears, hopes, the fun and the pain were shared, thereby enabling the group members to interact with each other and with their loved one more effectively. The groups themselves are a valuable tool in opening up new patterns of networking either pertaining to the life of the group or to home and local community based living experiences. In itself, the HIV infection crisis has become a powerful motivator for change on many levels for the 'significant others'.

Points for discussion

1. Discuss the range of feelings that may have to be faced up to by a relative or a partner of a person diagnosed as HIV positive.

2. Discuss the effect of the media coverage of AIDS issues on relatives or partners of people diagnosed as HIV positive.

3. In what ways can health and social services force the person suffering from HIV or AIDS into a more dependent role? How can services avoid this?

4. Assess the role of BRIDGE in relation to questions 1 - 3 above.

5. How do you 'bring back social networking'? Answer this question (a) in general terms and (b) in the specific context of the work of BRIDGE.

6. Assess the merits of a group work approach on the basis of the researcher's comments after attending an open session of the group at BRIDGE.

Reference

1. World Health Organisation (1988), *AIDS Prevention and Control.*

Chapter 6

The social worker as HIV health promoter

Previous chapters have demonstrated that in order appropriately to care for people with HIV and AIDS and encourage effective responses to the lifestyles challenges posed by HIV infection, all the efforts by individuals and organisations have to be orchestrated into agreed strategies where participation and harmonisation of effort are the key factors. It is argued that a social network approach will assist in such strategy developments by identifying the societal forces and social structures which must be harnessed and worked with to maximise opportunities or choice, despite HIV.

Health promotion

Before considering the role of the social worker as health promoter it is important to define what is meant by health promotion. It is helpful for there to be a wide ranging definition which embraces the changes required to be made both in the environment and by the individual in response to HIV infection. Health promotion principally means making healthy choices the easy choices. To achieve this, however, requires a combination of health education and intervention at a societal level by managers and policy makers as well as politicians designed to produce changes that are conducive to health. The following elements are the most important:

1. Action by the individual to prevent infection through avoidance of HIV risk behaviour.

2. Action by the individual with HIV to live a positively healthy life in order to prevent progression to AIDS.

3. Avoidance of victim-blaming and stigmatisation of people with HIV or AIDS. Victim blaming can neatly distance the rest of society from an infection which potentially affects everyone in Society.

4. Action by managers, policy makers and politicians to facilitate health options and HIV risk avoidance by individuals and groups.

5. The creation of a society in which individual members can make a contribution which leads to their feeling affirmed as people of worth. HIV infection feeds off anomie. Individuals feel alienated by virtue of their poor environment, unemployment, isolated social situation etc.

Health promotion within social services

For the social worker to take on board the role of health promotion, the profession has to begin by realising the tremendous untapped potential for this activity. Health promotion theoretically and practically involves all professions working within a community. It is argued, therefore, that social workers cannot ignore the health of their clients or the dis-ease of certain communities in which their clients live. Health influences people's lives to the extent that poor health creates social problems. Conversely, poor social conditions will influence the physical and mental health of the client. Therefore, it is essential that the social worker take on the important role of health promotion. To put all the eggs in the crisis-intervention basket is to run the risk of providing a lop-sided service to the client. In consequence, counselling both on a long term and short term basis must address those issues that surround the health of the individual and the health of the community, be those issues drug use (including smoking and alcohol use) sexual health, or HIV infection. It would be arrogant to confine the role of health promotion to social workers when staff at all levels of the organisation from director, Elected Members of committees (Councillors) to home helps have the potential for promoting the health of the community that they serve.

HIV health promotion within social services

The advent of HIV has seen the creation of a number of AIDS co-ordinator posts within social service organisations. These co-ordinators carry a key responsibility for the integration of HIV health promotion strategies into the basic fabric of social service delivery. To exercise this responsibility certain key tasks have to be carried out. These are:

1. Keeping the Elected Members and the director of the services aware of HIV and related issues (e.g., the need for localised drug misuse, prevention strategies, resources required to promote safer sex).

2. Liaison and networking with key others within the department (see *Figure 19*).

3. Liaison and networking with key others outwith the social service department (see *Figure 20*).

4. Provision of training for staff regarding HIV-AIDS. Liaison with local and national training resources can support 'in-house' training.

5. Consultancy service to individual social service staff working with clients living with HIV or AIDS in order to optimise the service given to the clients.

6. Liaison with key others in the authority (Personnel, Law and Administration Departments and trade unions) in order to prepare HIV-AIDS and drug policies for the authority.

7. Questioning attitudes and highlighting concerns about all aspects of HIV and AIDS held individually by staff members or collectively by bureaucracies.

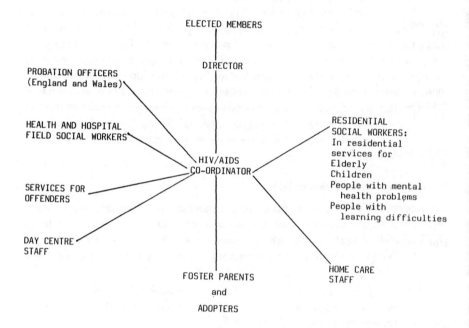

ELECTED MEMBERS

DIRECTOR

PROBATION OFFICERS
(England and Wales)

HEALTH AND HOSPITAL
FIELD SOCIAL WORKERS

HIV/AIDS
CO-ORDINATOR

RESIDENTIAL
SOCIAL WORKERS:
In residential
services for
Elderly
Children
People with mental
    health problems
People with
    learning difficulties

SERVICES FOR
OFFENDERS

DAY CENTRE
STAFF

FOSTER PARENTS
and
ADOPTERS

HOME CARE
STAFF

Fig. 19 - Liaison and networking within Social Services Departments

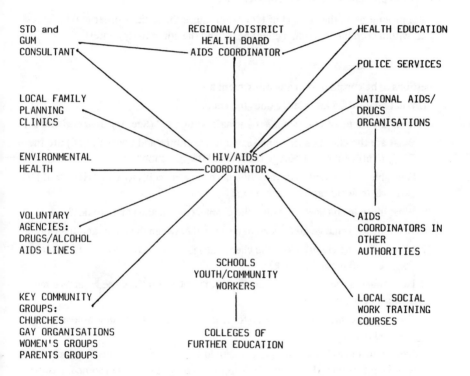

STD and
GUM
CONSULTANT

REGIONAL/DISTRICT
HEALTH BOARD
AIDS COORDINATOR

HEALTH EDUCATION

POLICE SERVICES

LOCAL FAMILY
PLANNING
CLINICS

NATIONAL AIDS/
DRUGS
ORGANISATIONS

ENVIRONMENTAL
HEALTH

HIV/AIDS
COORDINATOR

VOLUNTARY
AGENCIES:
DRUGS/ALCOHOL
AIDS LINES

AIDS
COORDINATORS IN
OTHER
AUTHORITIES

SCHOOLS
YOUTH/COMMUNITY
WORKERS

KEY COMMUNITY
GROUPS:
CHURCHES
GAY ORGANISATIONS
WOMEN'S GROUPS
PARENTS GROUPS

LOCAL SOCIAL
WORK TRAINING
COURSES

COLLEGES OF
FURTHER EDUCATION

Fig. 20 - Liaison and networking outside Social Services Departments

8. Promoting the consideration of HIV, safer sex and safer drug use as integral elements of any social work assessment.

9. Encouraging consideration and action by the department with regard to wider community and environmental issues that relate to HIV-AIDS prevention where the department can effectively intervene.

HIV health promotion - a social network model

Health promotion in the context of HIV will require the social worker making assessments within both the individual client home and the community context.

The individual home context

Questions to be considered in any assessment are:

1. What HIV-AIDS knowledge does the client have?

2. Does the client practice safer sex and safer drug use? (See *Appendices B* and *C*.)

3. What are the client's social and sexual relationships and how (if at all) are these likely to prevent or encourage the risk of HIV infection?

4. How able is the client to develop the necessary life skills to avoid HIV or, if HIV positive, to avoid repeated infection?

5. What lifestyle changes are within the client's control and what are not?

6. What lifestyle change goals need to be agreed between the client and the worker?

7. How well is the client? Does the client engage in any activities which puts health (physical and mental) at risk?

8. How aware is the client of the necessity for a nutritious balanced diet as a means of maximising immunity?

9. How does the client view the need for rest and relaxation and how able are they to rest and relax?

For those individuals living with HIV it should be stressed that the development of chronic HIV infection (ARC) and AIDS appear to be determined in some measure by the maintenance of as good a state of health as possible. The focus of work with individuals who have HIV or AIDS or who are at risk of infection should be on boosting the efficiency of their immune system functioning rather than on HIV *per se*. This may be achieved through approaches equated with holistic medicine (see *Appendix B*). Certain habits and lifestyles seem to have a negative effect on health in general and undermine immune functions in particular. These can be categorised as:

- stress.
- receptive anal intercourse (sperm is an immune supressive agent and damage to the lower gastro-intestinal tract can also be caused).
- the use of petrochemical-based lubricants for anal intercourse.

- the use of nitrates 'Poppers' as orgasm enhancers or anal sphincter relaxants.
- recurrent sexually transmitted diseases.
- the use of antibiotics and other drugs to deal with infections which can lower immunity.
- the development of infections (ie thrush, herpes) leading to additional immune stress.

Development of HIV, ARC and AIDS.

It is important to caution against such lifestyles being necessarily associated with gay men, although they may be more prevalent within that community.

The key elements of assessment of individuals can be remembered by using the acronym SENSES:

- Stress and life management skills
- Emotional well being
- Nutrition and diet
- Safer drug use (including alcohol and nicotine)
- Exercise and relaxation
- Safer sex

It is important for social workers and HIV counsellors to remember that if the focus of their work with the client is around the area of personal responsibility for health, then the key to successful intervention is careful timing. It is important that the client feels challenged by the goal of maximising immunity and not overwhelmed either by the task or the consideration of HIV. It is also essential that counselling should be done within the context of positive prescriptive advice rather than negative messages. The promotion and reinforcement of individual and group behaviour change is done better by such messages as:

'Dress up your fantasies - wear a condom'

rather than:

'Don't have unprotected sex'

The home context

The role of families, loved ones and partners of people living with HIV and AIDS is crucial. They too will have many attitudes and concerns in respect of HIV. Health promotion means involving them in the health goals. By example and encouragement family and partners can support their loved one who has HIV or is at risk of infection by virtue of their own lifestyles. The model for assessment already outlined can easily be adapted to the home context.

The community context

The social environment for HIV prevention must be one that is highly conducive towards, and supportive of, positive HIV prevention strategies. The 'social marketing' approach to health promotion has highlighted the benefits of involving target groups within the community in joint ventures aimed at achieving not only HIV prevention behaviour outcomes but also the provision of resources which can facilitate healthy choices. The social worker and community worker are potential catalysts in achieving health promotion goals by working with the existing community networks. However, communities will only exercise a responsible commitment to HIV health promotion goals when they (like the individual) are empowered to address and manage a threat such as HIV and AIDS. They will only be able to address the issue when they are in a sense 'healthy'. To respond to the challenges of HIV and AIDS, a healthy community has to listen, react, respond to the changes that HIV requires and utilise policy makers, politicians, service provides, service users and their families in the process. Such a response has been defined as 'Community Competence' or the ability to respond to the public health threat of HIV in a way that enables the community to prepare for the next threat.[1]

For social workers to adopt a community perspective to health promotion in respect of HIV they will need to answer some of the following questions:

1. What is the nature of the community on which to target? (Target groups for health change should be identified. These may be drug users, sex industry workers (prostitutes), the Gay community, the local prison, pubs and clubs, church groups, political groupings etc.)

2. What formal and informal systems of networking already exist in the community which can be utilised for HIV health promotion?

3. What does the community already know about HIV and AIDS and has it already formulated any action strategies?

4. Have there been instances of reactions in the community which may be counterproductive to HIV health promotion (e.g., attitudes to prostitutes, needle exchanges, condom availability in youth clubs)?

5. Are HIV prevention measures available and accessible (e.g., needle exchange schemes, chemists that will sell/collect needles and syringes, chemists/supermarkets selling condoms, condoms in public toilets/pubs etc)?

6. Do facilities exist that will help promote healthy and nutritious diets (shops, health food shops, etc.)?

7. What facilities exist that will help promote rest and relaxation (clubs, swimming baths, leisure and community centres, football, tennis and other sports facilities)?

8. What facilities exist for the promotion of good health in the community (medical and paramedical services, Community Health Councils etc.)?

9. Where is it and where is it not within the control of the community to affect health choices and options?

10. What HIV health promotion policies and strategies can be developed with and by the community?

Finally, the political will to provide resources must be harnessed through consultation. Without this political will, health providers, users of services and the community in general will struggle badly in its attempts to ensure an effective community response to HIV and AIDS.

The assessment of individual, home and community responses to HIV can be shown diagramatically as in *Figure 21*.

Examples

Using the models outlined, two HIV health promotion approaches in different communities are briefly described:

1. HIV health promotion within a prison.

2. HIV health promotion with sex industry workers.

Health promotion within a prison

The AIDS co-ordinator targeted a local prison for HIV health promotion. The objectives were fourfold:

1. To promote HIV health education amongst inmates and prison staff.

2. To develop the skills of the social work team in providing pre-test counselling, post-test follow up, drugs and sex risk counselling.

3. To examine with the prison staff general care of inmates who were HIV positive. Prescribing policies, general health care, diet, opportunities to relax or take physical recreation were considered.

4. To prepare the ground for voluntary organisations providing a buddying service or specialised drugs counselling.

To achieve this, an introductory approach was made to the Prison Governor enclosing details of an HIV leaflet prepared by and for inmates in another prison. The Governor then called a multidisciplinary meeting at which the following were present:

Governor, deputy and assistant governor, medical officer, nurse officer, psychologist, social workers and AIDS co-ordinator. Chaplaincy and psychiatric services were not able to be present but were informed.

As a result of the meeting the following targets were agreed:

1. Rolling training programme on HIV and AIDS (using Home Office video) for prison staff to be organised by training Governor and AIDS co-ordinator.

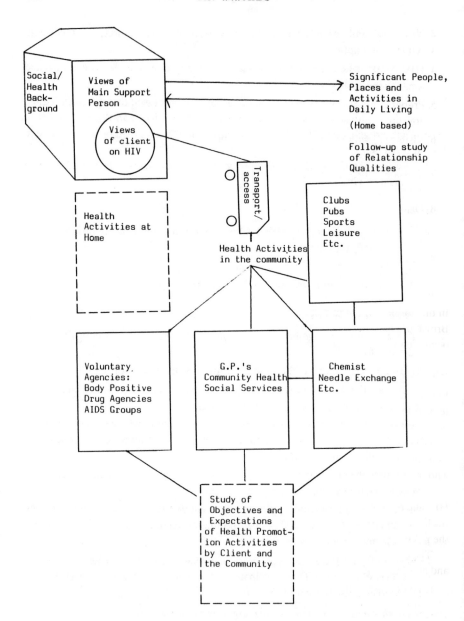

Fig. 21 - Information components required for HIV health promotion in the Home and Community context

2. HIV-AIDS leaflets distributed to prison staff for information.

3. AIDS leaflet to be adapted by inmates for own use through art class project.

4. HIV-AIDS programme to be organised by AIDS co-ordinator for inmates using small group technique and videos etc.

5. Preparation of social work team to provide pre-test counselling and post-test follow up.

6. Visits to identified inmates who had requested drugs counselling prior to their discharge.

7. Consideration of special dietary needs of inmates with known HIV or Hepatitis B infection.

8. Discussion with community dietician of prison diet and need for vitamin supplements, etc., where it was found that a special diet might have discriminatory knock-on effects and cause management problems for the whole prison.

9. Detailed discussion of difficult issues, e.g. drugs in the prison, situational homosexuality.

10. Agreement to follow up meetings at regular intervals to monitor progress.

In the absence of the likelihood of free needles and condoms being made available in British prisons, it was nevertheless felt that the described initiatives went some way to beginning HIV health promotion in this particular prison.

HIV health promotion with sex industry workers* and their clients

In undertaking this work, it was recognised from the beginning that targeting male and female sex industry workers in any particular city should not be done from the standpoint that they were, by definition, a high risk group of people who were a major threat to the general population as likely carriers of the HIV virus. Health promotion was carried out on the basis that these workers were probably at increased risk from their clients who might offer greater financial reward for unsafe sexual services. It was recognised that sex industry workers would probably on the whole be quite knowledgeable about HIV and other sexually transmitted diseases. A major concern, however, was that where the financing of an injection drug habit was equated with the needs, for sex industry work the risks of HIV infection were greater.

The objectives of the health promotion work undertaken by the AIDS co-ordinator and another social worker were:

1. To determine the nature and extent of the sex industry work in the city. (On the street, in saunas, escort agencies, from hotels, etc.)

---

*The term 'Sex Industry Workers' is becoming more commonly used, often replacing the word 'Prostitute' - a term carrying as it does many depreciatory connotations - Ed.

2. To ascertain how much the sex industry workers knew about HIV and AIDS and pass on information and advice accordingly.

3. To assess whether knowledge about HIV had led to behaviour change.

4. To promote the practice of safer sex by the provision of free condoms.

5. To determine the extent that the use of alcohol and other drugs might influence the non-practice of safer sex.

6. To assess the extent that the sex industry work was related to financial stress (in particular financial stress caused by the need to maintain a drug habit).

7. To determine how much pressure there was on the sex industry workers to engage in unsafe sex for higher financial rewards.

8. To determine how aware the clients of the sex industry workers were of HIV and AIDS and whether this awareness had influenced their requests for sexual services.

9. To investigate the role potential of sex industry workers as health educators of their clients.

10. By identifying needs, to determine the services that would be needed for the continuation of HIV health promotion amongst sex industry workers and their clients.

To achieve these objectives the workers had to spend several months at street level gaining the confidence of the men and women engaged in the sex industry. Initially, the social workers were seen as 'authority' who might be a threat to the industry, but after a period of testing out, they came to be seen as helpful (advice, literature, dealing with other non-related problems, providers of condoms) and 'on our side'. The social workers asked the sex industry workers to complete an anonymous confidential questionnaire which could be returned if they wished. This questionnaire covered the following areas:

1. Basic details of age, sex, sex industry work in other cities in Britain and abroad.

2. Knowledge of HIV and where obtained.

3. Contact with sexually transmitted diseases (STD) and Genito Urinary Medicine (GUM) clinics.

4. Whether the sex industry worker had been tested for HIV. (How often? Result?)

5. Whether the sex industry worker had been subject to violence and if so from whom?

6. Attitudes to safer sex.

7. Whether the sexual practices with casual clients differed in a way from those practised with partners or 'regular' clients?

8. The use of drugs (including alcohol).

9. Information and services identified by the sex industry workers as being needed.

10. Any other comments the workers wished to make.

An attempt was made to evaluate the extent of the sex industry by identifying places 'off the street' where the industry could be located or where casual sexual encounters could be expected. These included saunas, hotels, pubs and clubs, public toilets, escort agencies. The strategies for safer sex promotion differed according to the location identified.

The social workers undertaking the health promotion networked with a variety of organisations including:

- consultant and HIV counsellor at STD clinic
- family planning services
- local police
- local drug agency and social services staff
- gay community representatives (Gay Switchboard)
- local AIDS line
- other workers in other British cities engaged in similar work

Contacts with pub owners in the area in which the sex industry work was undertaken, and also taxi services, were targeted for information because of their practice of touting for sex industry workers on behalf of clients in hotels.

During the time the social workers were involved in their HIV health promotion work, in response to community pressure the local police had a major clamp down on the sex industry workers and their clients. As a result contact with the sex industry workers became harder to maintain, especially as there was a geographical diffusion of the industry and a move more into escort agency type situations.

Points for discussion

1. How can a social network approach assist with HIV health promotion?

2. Discuss the process of targetting a health education project.

3. Discuss community attitudes to the sex industry, drugs and safer sex in the context of health education.

4. In what ways may the social worker's personal beliefs affect his approach to health eduation issues in this field, such as safer sex?

5. In what ways can the social worker take account of the possible religious beliefs of the client concerning, for example, attitudes to sex and marriage?

6. Discuss the place of political involvement in HIV health education.

7. Consider the importance of healthy eating as part of healthy living. What are some of the difficulties in effectively promoting healthy eating?

8. Discuss the application of health education principles and practices to (a) the prison project and (b) the sex industry workers and clients project.

Reference

1. Scottish Health Education Group/World Health Organisation (1984), *Health Promotion an Overview*.

Chapter 7

Looking to the future

The spread of HIV and AIDS has been well described as a 'catastrophe in slow motion'.[1] In the past four years the number of AIDS cases worldwide reported to the World Health Organisation has increased more than fifteen-fold. The number of cases of HIV infection can only be guessed at but it is thought there are at least 50 people infected with HIV for every case of AIDS. A cure may be at least ten years away and an effective vaccine is not yet available. Such is the scenario of the worldwide HIV/AIDS pandemic which is slowly unfolding. The effects of HIV and AIDS however, go beyond mere health statistics when the economic, social, cultural and political aspects of, and reactions to, the infection are considered. It is not the purpose of this book to engage in political debate save to say that prevention programmes and HIV intervention strategies will not happen without the necessary political will and financial wherewithal. If thinly disguised prejudices about so called 'risk groups' or risk practices are allowed to colour judgements and influence the provision of resources, it is safe to say that the virus will continue its slow and insidious spread worldwide.

AIDS has to be placed firmly on the agenda for action by health and social service authorities and by local communities so that intervention programmes can be devised and carried out. It is recognised that broad brush public information campaigns have limited value in producing the rapid or even sustained behaviour changes that are required to prevent HIV infection. In consequence, to confront the issues surrounding HIV and AIDS requires differential approaches to be adapted to the complex social problems surrounding HIV and AIDS. It is argued that the social network approach as described in this book is one such method which can facilitate a better understanding of these social problems before action plans are identified and targeted. However, before a social network approach can be adopted as a method of working by social service departments, it is essential that HIV and AIDS are legitimised as a valid and appropriate area of work for these departments to be involved in. Up until now the prospects for such a legitimisation have not looked good. Social work as a profession has been notoriously indifferent to many of the elements which come together to form the AIDS reality, in particular, those associated with drug misuse and sexuality. Although HIV and AIDS is a relatively new issue for social workers in historical terms there is no reason why these workers should feel de-skilled if they incorporate the new knowledge into their existing therapeutic intervention skills. As has been recently pointed out by the

British Association of Social Workers in its publication *HIV/AIDS - A Social Work Perspective*, social workers have contributed to the care of people suffering from incurable illnesses and have worked with people who are stigmatised (e.g. the person with a mental illness, the child in residential care) for many years. Yet issues around drug users have been mainly hived off to a specialist worker and issues around sexuality largely ignored. Gay men, sex industry workers, drug misusers (of all drugs) have had a notoriously patchy service from social care authorities, if they have received one at all. HIV and AIDS have helped to highlight the inadequacies and inequalities in not only health systems but also the social care systems. If the social care system has a problem empathising with, and caring for, those people who, by virtue of risk behaviour, are at risk or have contracted HIV, then this fact will be remorsely highlighted. HIV and AIDS have also shaken complacencies in that social carers cannot assume that everything is all right unless there is a crisis. For example, HIV means the necessity for departments to validate and take responsibility for the safer sexual expression of the residents in their care, be they children, those with learning difficulties, the physically handicapped or the elderly. At the end of the day there is no reason why social service departments and social workers in particular, should not play key roles in implementing two of the main strands of the World Health Organisation AIDS Strategy namely:

- to prevent HIV infection
- to reduce the personal and social impact of HIV infection and to care for those already infected with HIV or who have AIDS

Enough is now known on how to prevent HIV and since it is the behaviour of individuals which is responsible for most HIV transmission, the social work profession must do all it can do to inform and educate about the ways to prevent infection. Risk behaviour must be modified as much as possible through the practice of safer sex and safer drug use. In order to do this specific target groups and individuals need to be identified for information giving and education. Such a process goes side by side with the counselling required to support and strengthen individual groups and communities in making longer term shifts in behaviour and attitudes to HIV risk. Whilst counselling is often a more personal and intimate process whereby the individual can find information and support during the processes of behavioural change, it is important to widen the context through consideration of family, social and community networks which, by necessity, will shape and influence any counselling goals. It has been demonstrated that the social network approach facilitates this consideration.

To meet the second objective of the World Health Organisation requires social service organisations to provide care for people living with AIDS and those infected with HIV and not ill. Such care should be sensitive, compassionate, unconditional and aimed at assisting the person living with HIV and AIDS to live as healthy and as stress free a life as possible. Care should be independence creating and not dependence disabling. Care should be located as much as possible within the mainstream of departmental life

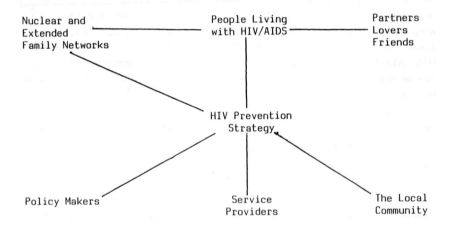

Fig. 22 - A model for integrative planning

and not sited discreetly at the periphery. People with HIV and AIDS have been marginalised enough. To assess ways in which this care can be assimilated into the social fabric of the department as well as the social fabric of the community, the social network approach can usefully be used by studying the interaction between:

- the person cared for, their family, their partners and friends.
- the people providing the care.
- the context in which the care is provided.

Making connections

To enable individuals and communities to live positively requires an integrative approach which takes full cognisance of the social context in which this potentially life threatening disease is spreading and will continue to spread. The value of the social network approach lies in its ability to facilitate the integration. The integration may be on a personal level or within a group or community context as the main issues pertinant to HIV and AIDS are assimilated and worked through - issues such as living well, sexuality, disease, disability, death. The integration may also be on a strategic level as evidenced by planning HIV prevention strategies.

A model for integrative planning is represented in *Figure 22*. On whatever level, the essential factor is the need to assess and develop linkages and networks. To do so is to:

- develop potential standards of care for people living with HIV and AIDS
- enable the person living with HIV and AIDS to be empowered and take control over the direction of his or her life.
- work towards achieving a healthier, integrated environment and community.
- develop and enhance good social work practice.

The Director of the World Health Organisation AIDS programme, Dr J. Mann, stated in 1988:

'We are still in the early phases of a global epidemic whose first decade gives every reason for concern about the future.'[2]

Looking to the HIV future, therefore, means recognising the linkages between individuals and societies. A social network approach facilitates the understanding of these linkages because HIV and AIDS as a disease process can be challenged. The challenge is as much about the approaches to the combat as it is about the nature of the battle.

Reference

1. Sontag, Susan. *AIDS and its Metaphors*. Review in the *Observer* Newspaper. April 1989.
2. World Health Organisation, (1988), *AIDS Prevention and Control*, Pergamon Press.

Bibliography

(1987), *AIDS and HIV. Information for Foster Parents*, National Foster Care Association Publications.

(1987), *The Implication of AIDS for Children in Care*, British Agencies for Adoption and Fostering Publications.

(1987), *Living with AIDS - A Guide to Survival by People With AIDS*, Frontliners.

Aggleton P., and Homans, H., (1988), *Social Aspects of AIDS*, The Falmer Press.

Aggleton, P., Hart, G., and Davies, P., (eds), (1989), *AIDS Social Representations, Social Practices*, The Falmer Press.

Aggleton, P., Homans, H., et al., (1989), *AIDS Scientific and Social Issues*, Churchill Livingstone.

Bamford, M., Gaitley, R., and Miller, R., (eds), (1988), *HIV - AIDS. A Social Work Perspective*, British Association of Social Workers Publications.

Chaitow, L., and Martin, S., (1988), *A World Without AIDS*, Thorsons Publication Group.

Daniels, V.G., Dr., (1987), *AIDS. The Acquired Immune Deficiency Syndrome* (2nd edition), MTP Press.

Gordon, P., and Mitchell, L., (1988), *Safer Sex*, Faber and Faber.

Hockings, J., (1988), *Walking The Tightrope (Living Positively, with AIDS, ARC and HIV)*, Gate Centre Publications.

Miller, D., Dr., (1987), *Living with AIDS*, MacMillan.

Richardson, D., (1987), *Women and the AIDS Crisis*, Pandora.

Robertson, R., Dr., (1987), *Heroin, AIDS and Society*, Hodder and Stoughton.

Seed, P., (1989), *Introducing Network Analysis in Social Work*, Jessica Kingsley Publishers.

Spence, C., (1986), *AIDS Time to Reclaim our Power*, Lifestory Press.

Tatchell, P., (1986), *AIDS - A Guide to Survival*, Gay Mens Press.

Wilkinson, G., (1987), *Working with Gay Men with AIDS*, Sussex AIDS Line.

World Health Organisation, (1988), *AIDS Prevention and Control*, Pergamon Press.

The meaning of HIV and AIDS

To assist in the understanding of the terminology used in this book, a brief synopsis of the relevant information is given. For a more detailed discussion of the scientific and epidemiological aspects of AIDS please consult those titles referred to in the bibliography.

What is meant by AIDS and HIV?

AIDS is the abbreviated form used to describe the Acquired Immune Deficiency Syndrome.

ACQUIRED - The infection HIV is caught. It is not inherited.

IMMUNE DEFICIENCY - The body's immune system (its primary defence system against illness) has become deficient due to being undermined by HIV.

SYNDROME - The presence of one or more specific illnessess and cancers which have taken the opportunity (hence they are often referred to as 'opportunistic') to develop and become potentially life threatening due to the collapse of the immune system. These diseases would rarely affect people whose immune systems were working well and one or more have to be present before a diagnosis of AIDS can be made. All other causes of immune deficiency (e.g. Immune Suppressive Drugs) have to be discounted.

HIV

The virus which can lead to AIDS is called HIV which is short for Human Immunodeficiency Virus. Two strains of the virus, HIV 1 and HIV 2, have been identified. On entering the body the virus attacks the white cells (known as 'T4' helper cells) which are responsible for activating and co-ordinating the body's response to infectious diseases. Eventually, the cells can become so immobilised that the body is unable to resist infection. It is at this point that certain infections associated with chronic HIV infection (also known as ARC or AIDS Related Complex) and AIDS may develop.

HIV is a composite term adopted by WHO in 1985 for the believed causative virus which had been formerly known as:

AIDS Associated Retrovirus (ARV) or

Lymphadenopathy Associated Virus (LAV) or

Human 'T' Cell Lymphotropic Virus Type 3 (HTLV 3).

It is essential to understand that being infected with HIV and having a diagnosis of AIDS is not one and the same. It is for this reason that phrases as 'The AIDS virus', 'The AIDS test', 'The AIDS sufferer' are misleading and detrimentally inaccurate because of the linkages some people make between AIDS and inevitable illness and death. Accurate references to HIV can often be a springboard to promote realistic hope for the person who is living with the virus and manifestly not 'dying of AIDS'.

The clinical sequelae of HIV Infection

The recent definitions used by the Centre for Disease Control, Atlanta, offer a flexible classification which mirrors the uncertainties and ever widening clinical spectrum of HIV and AIDS. The definition identifies four basic outcomes of HIV infection.

1. Acute infection

Although antibodies are produced by the immune response to HIV these are ineffective in preventing the virus replicating and infecting other T4 helper cells. Within a few weeks of exposure to HIV the person infected may experience a mononucleosis type illness (similar to glandular fever) with symptoms of aching, rashes and swollen lymph glands. Transient meningitis and neuropathy also have been very occasionally noted as indicative of an attack by HIV on the functioning of the central nervous system.

2. Symptomatic infection

Most people who have been infected with HIV are unaware of the fact as they show no symptoms. Their blood and sexual fluids are, however, potentially infectious, especially in the latter stages of AIDS. It is not known how many people with HIV will go on to develop symptoms associated with PGL, ARC or AIDS. The mean time between HIV and the development of AIDS may be eight years but the discussion of averages and percentages is of little help diagnostically or therapeutically in projecting the illness career of a person with HIV.

There are indicators, however, that co-factors may be very significant in delaying or hastening the onset of chronic HIV infection and AIDS. On the positive side the main factor appears to be the living of as healthy and stress-free a life as possible. On the negative side, there are factors such as repeated HIV infection, the presence of other recurring sexually transmitted diseases and the continued use of immune suppressive drugs such as opiates, amphetamines, nitrates ('poppers') and alcohol.

3. Persistent generalised lymphadenopathy (PGL)

PGL is characterised by a persistent (at least 3 months) swelling of the lymph nodes in two distinctly separate sites of the body (neck, armpits) other than the groin. As it is quite common for a person's lymph glands to swell in response to infection, for a diagnosis of PGL to be made the swelling has to be unexplained, non-tender and in excess of 1 centimetre in diameter. Other symptoms may accompany the swelling including fevers, night sweats, diarrhoea, marked loss of body weight, bouts of unexplained tiredness and acne.

4. Other more significant diseases

Significant of a systematic collapse of the immune system are conditions known as:.

AIDS Related Complex (ARC).

Additional to those symptoms mentioned under PGL, other symptoms may be present, for example, cutaneous staphylococcal infections, minor skin infection (herpes zoster ('shingles'), eczema, folliculitis), and oral candida (thrush). Therapeutic treatment with antiviral and antiretroviral drugs may slow down any development to AIDS.

AIDS

AIDS is a syndrome, a kaleisdoscope of disorders and opportunistic infections which may be focalised or disseminated throughout the body.

Some of the opportunistic infections and cancers commonly associated with a diagnosis of AIDS are:

Protozoal infections

- Pneumocystis Carinii Pneumonia (PCP) (persistent breathlessness on exertion with fever, chest pains and a dry non productive cough).
- Cryptosporidium Enteritis (bouts of persistent diarrhoea which is hard to control by conventional therapies, leading to severe weight loss).
- Toxoplasmosis (disseminated infection lymph nodes and blood).

Bacterial infections

- various Mycobacterium infections, including tuberculosis, avium intracellular - leading to a disseminated infection involving the lungs, spleen, lymphatic system and other body organs.
- Shigella (affecting the intestine leading to diarrhoea).

Fungal infections

- Candida Oesaphagitis (*Thrush*) (the mouth, gullet and stomach may be affected, leading to sores and severe discomfort in eating and swallowing).

- Cryptococcal infections (pulmonary generalised infections - usually manifested by the wearing away of the central, sympathetic and para sympathetic nervous system - can lead to meningitis).
- Histoplasmosis (leading to pneumonia and disseminated infections).

Viral infections

- Cytomegalovirus (CMV) (ulceration in the gut by a herpes type virus which can also affect the central nervous system).
- Herpes Simplex Virus (ulcerated sores in the mouth, genitals, buttocks - can also affect the central nervous system.)
- Epstein-Barr Virus (disseminated infection of blood, liver, brain, lymph nodes).

Cancers

- Tumours associated with a diagnosis of AIDS.
- Kaposis Sarcoma (KS) (A rare aggressive skin cancer presenting as purple blotches on skin surface, palate of the mouth, sometimes in the gastrointestinal and respiratory systems. This cancer appears to be more commonly found in gay men than injecting drug users.).
- Lymphomas (cancers of the lymphatic system - non-Hodgkins Lymphoma, Hodgkins Disease, Burkitts Lymphoma). Tumours in the brain and central nervous system.

Neurological disorders

- Any definition of AIDS must now take account of the subtle damage which can happen to the brain and the central nervous system as a result of HIV infection. Presentation of this damage (HIV encephalopathy, cryptococcus meningitis, spinal cord and peripheral nerve infection) can lead to a loss of body co-ordination, a marked diminution in intellectual functioning, behavioural disorders and early dementia. Again it should be stressed that although these presentations have been identified they are not necessarily a *sine qua non* of an AIDS diagnosis. The prospects of this might cause alarm to people living with HIV and AIDS as well as to their carers.
- It should also be noted that in drug users it is often clinically difficult to distinguish between AIDS-associated dementia and drug induced encephalopathy.

Treatments for HIV and AIDS

Although HIV and AIDS cannot be cured, antiretroviral and antiviral drugs have been used with noticeably beneficial effect in treatment. These drugs ideally have to:

1. Stop or slow HIV virus production in the 'T' cells.
2. Boost the immune system functioning and cell ratio levels.

3. Cross the blood/brain barrier in order to deal with the viral damage to the central nervous system and brain.

4. Be relatively non-toxic as they will have to be taken for life.

Of the drugs developed the most well known are:.

Zidovidine or **'AZT'** (*'Retrovir'* - *trade name*) (an antiretroviral drug which may have toxic side effects leading to bone marrow disease, anaemia, insomnia - regular blood transfusions may therefore be indicated). AZT used in conjunction with Dideoxycytidine is a promising current therapy.

Naltrexone (a relatively cheap and low toxicity drug which leads to an increase in the body's level of endorphins and enkephalins, both of which appear to assist immune functioning and the communications between the immune system and the central nervous system).

AL 721 (an egg yolk high potency lecithin anti-cancer remedy developed by scientists in Israel. The drug (which can be made extremely cheaply using products found in most health stores) appears to help cell membranes to become resistant to viral attacks. There has been considerable medical controversy over the use of AL 721 as an effective antiviral agent, but the drug has been shown to have been of considerable help for some people with AIDS. Results from the use of AL 721 are still very preliminary but nevertheless cautiously encouraging.).

Symptom control

There are a number of drugs which appear to be effective in controlling the symptoms of the opportunistic infections associated with ARC and AIDS. If the therapy begins early enough most people who are infected do recover:

Co-trimaxozole (Septrin) **Nebulised Pentamidine** }	for the treatment of 'PCP'
Sulphadiazine	for the treatment of toxoplasmosis
Nystatin **Clotrimazole** }	for the treatment of candida (thrush)
Ganciclovir	for the treatment of cytomegalovirus (CMV)

Radiotherapy, chemotherapy and alpha-interferon are also used for the treatment of tumours associated with AIDS.

Holistic health and complementary medicines

Holistic approaches to health, focusing as they do on the healing of the whole person (mind, body, spirit) and not just on HIV and AIDS, seem to have major benefits in maximising immunity. By taking a positive interest in being healthy, the person with HIV (and indeed all of us) can prevent disease development and stimulate the body's natural processes of healing. Holistic treatment involves:

1. The use of conventional medicines.

2. The use of complementary medicines (see list).

3. The use of self help skills (see list).

The range of approaches and therapies which can be explored are:

Complementary medicine	Self help
Homeopathic medicines	Breathing and relaxation techniques
Herbalism	Meditation
Acupuncture	Biofeedback
Acupressure	Positive visualisation
Hydrotherapy	Yoga
Hypnotherapy	Aromatherapy
Naturopathy	Appropriate physical exercise
Reflexology	Autogenic training
Emotional expression and spiritual enquiry	Diet (particularly increased intake of Vitamin C)

Whichever approach or combination of approaches are adopted, the bottom line must be the recognition that people with HIV and AIDS are not passive patients subject to the ravages of the virus HIV. They are people with the capacity to reorganise their lives by living a positively healthy life, thereby benefiting body, mind and spirit and, in particularly, the immune system in the process.

Transmission of HIV

The virus has been isolated in various concentrations in all body fluids, particularly blood and sexual fluids, but apart from breast milk (and theoretically urine) there are thought to be no risks of transmission of HIV by tears, saliva, or sweat. In consequence, there is no evidence that HIV can be transmitted by kissing, coughing, sneezing, body contact, cutlery and crockery, towels and linen, or via food, pets, insects and mosquitoes, sharing communal bathing and washing facilities or from toilets.

Three routes for transmission of HIV have been identified:

1. Sexual transmission

Through penetrative sexual intercourse (vaginally and anally) with an infected person (male or female) without using a condom and leading to an exchange of sexual body fluids (seminal fluids, vaginal and cervical secretions). The evidence regarding genito-oral sex HIV transmission remains unclear but should be regarded as possible. (For a more detailed discussion on 'Safer sex' see *Appendix B*).

2. Blood and blood products

Through an inoculation of blood infected with HIV. This is primarily through:
- a transfusion of blood infected with HIV.
- a blood component (ie blood-plasma factor 8, factor 9) infected with HIV.
- the sharing by drug users of drug injecting equipment which has been infected with HIV. (For a more detailed discussion on 'Safer drug use' see *Appendix C*).
- HIV can also be transmitted by organ and tissue transplants.

Medical injections using non-sterile equipment and other activities involving the piercing of the skin by needle (i.e. tattooing, ear piercing, acupuncture, electrolysis) are also theoretically potential routes for HIV transmission.

In Britain, Northern America and Europe blood donations, blood products, organ, semen, and tissue donations have been routinely screened for a number of years. As it takes three months for the antibodies to HIV to show after infection (a period called 'the window of infection') there remains a one-in-a-million risk of infection by these donations. Sensitive tests for the HIV antigen (a component of the virus which can be detected before antibody reaction) are being urgently developed to add to the range screening to eliminate transmission of HIV. Screening processes have also been modified to detect HIV 2 (a recently identified viral strain of HIV which is transmitted in similar ways to HIV 1).

3. Transmission from mother to child

A mother with HIV can transmit the virus to her unborn foetus cross-placentally. A few cases world wide have now indicated the possibility of transmission via breast feeding. Medical controversy about transmission during the birth process or by a particular method of birth delivery has made it difficult to determine categorically that these routes for transmission are indicated, but for the time being it should be assumed that these are possibilities.

The epidemiology of HIV/AIDS

The World Health Organisation have divided the epidemiological considerations of HIV/AIDS into three separate but interdependent epidemics:
1. Infection with HIV.

2. The disease AIDS.

3. The response to HIV and AIDS as determined on social, cultural, economic and political levels.

1. Infection with HIV

There is little reliable information available on the global prevalence of HIV infection. The World Health Organisation has estimated (1988) a prevalence rate of 5 - 10 million. In Britain by the beginning of July 1988, 8,794 actual cases had been reported as a result of testing and, of those tested, 'guestimates' of HIV positive ranged between 30,000 and 50,000. In England and Wales the majority (84%) are gay and bisexual men while in Scotland the majority (54%) are injecting drug users. All figures should, however, be treated with caution given known sociological factors such as population mobility. Major ethical and legal problems have arisen around suggestions for national serosurveillance surveys. On the whole these are seen as socially and politically unacceptable. The World Health Organisation has determined three separate patterns of HIV infection:.

A. Pattern I Countries (Americas, Europe)

Mostly gay and bisexual men are infected but injecting drug use spread of HIV is likely to attain greater prominence in the future. This may lead to an increase in the number of heterosexuals infected with HIV and an increased risk of materno-foetal transmission.

B. Pattern II Countries (Afro-Caribbean)

HIV transmission is predominantly heterosexual. Equal numbers of men and women are infected. In these countries the transfusion of HIV infected blood remains a problem for public health although testing and screening facilities are rapidly being developed.

C. Pattern III Countries (Russia, Asia, Far East)

The prevalence of HIV reported infection is still low and involves sexual transmission as well as the use of infected blood and blood transfusions. There is evidence that HIV is increasing in these countries.

Eventually, these three patterns may blend together. As safe blood and blood products along with infection control procedures for skin piercing practices becomes the norm worldwide, most HIV transmission will become sexual and perinatal as well as being the result of the sharing of infected drug equipment amongst drug users. *For this reason effective HIV prevention strategies must target everyone who could potentially engage in risk behaviour.*

2. AIDS

In January 1988, 75,392 cases of fully expressed AIDS were reported from 130 countries. By June 1988 this figure had risen to 100,400 cases from 138 countries. Delays in reporting and underreporting suggest that by mid-1988 a more realistic figure for those with AIDS worldwide would be 170,000 cases. 75% of the cases reported were in the Americas (primarily the North), 12% in Europe, and 12% in Afro-Caribbean countries. (Not all countries of the world are included in these figures.)

3. The response to AIDS

The World Health Organisation has pointed out that the future impact of AIDS will be seen on health care systems, national economies and demographic patterns primarily because 90% of cases of HIV and AIDS are among young adults and infants. The social impact of HIV and AIDS also has the potential for a marked impact on the possible progression of the epidemic, particularly in such areas as:.

1. The level and extent of behaviour change in response to the risk from practices associated with HIV and AIDS.

2. The stigma attached to those with HIV and AIDS.

3. The dysfunctional social effects associated with 'controlling deviants'.

4. The heavy responsibilities HIV and AIDS has placed on families, partners and caretakers of people living with the virus.

5. Health care planning needs associated with HIV and AIDS.

Appendix B

Safer sex

If a couple have had a monogamous totally faithful sexual relationship with each other, the risks of HIV infection will have been eliminated. Sometimes, however, this is a big 'if' and it is unwise to make assumptions, as many people within or embarking on a sexual relationship often find it hard to talk about sex to each other.

Human sexual knowledge, human sexual predilections and values, and human sexual error all make it imperative to talk about safer sex and unsafe sex in the context of HIV infection. The yardstick to adopt when considering the level of HIV transmission risk in any given sexual activity is relatively straightforward. Any sexual activity which allows body fluids (blood, seminal and vaginal fluid, cervical secretions) to enter another person (through orifices, cuts, mucosal surface lining) should always be considered unsafe.

It is appreciated that HIV has not yet been shown to be transmitted via faeces or urine although other viruses (e.g. cytomegalovirus (CMV) and hepatitis) have been transmitted in these ways. It is recommended that sexual activities which could lead to the transmission of other viruses by the same routes as HIV be also considered unsafe.

The options for safer sex

Human beings can enjoy safer sex in a wide variety of pleasurable ways which do not necessarily involve the penetration of the human body. Provided that these activities meet the yardstick already outlined they can be regarded as unlikely to lead to HIV infection. Health educators should therefore encourage people to be careful but inventive in their sexual lives and help the breakdown of any awkwardnesses that may be felt when discussing sexual practices and sexual attitudes.

In the context of HIV and other sexually transmitted diseases, it is important to remember that in any new relationship each partner will potentially inherit the sexual past history of the other. It is impossible to tell whether someone is, or has been, infected with HIV. Therefore it is best to assume this possibility and practice safer sex according to those activities which minimise the risk of infection. In discussing those sexual activities which may or may not lead to HIV certain categories can be used. It is recognised that it is not possible to be totally definitive and that there may be an element of overlap between the categories.

Unsafe sex

Vaginal and anal intercourse without a condom.

Any sexual activity which draws blood.

Fisting (fist-fucking - insertion of the finger, hand, wrist or arm into the anus and vaginal areas can lead to bleeding and be very unsafe, especially if accompanied by intercourse. A barrier such as a rubber glove or finger stall will cut down the risk).

Sharing sex toys, dildos, etc.

Using a douche and enema for washing out the vaginal and anal areas before or after sex (enemas remove the protective mucosal coating of the anus and vagina making them more vulnerable to infection; the practice also forces any infection higher in the body).

Risky sex

Urinating or defacating on your partner ('golden showers', 'water sports', 'skat').

Oral sex (man to man, man to woman, woman to man, woman to woman). The gums, mouth, penis and vaginal areas may have small cuts and other infections. Ejaculation should take place outside the mouth or with a dry and flavoured condom used as appropriate. Where there is menstrual blood present ('rainbow kissing') the risks are likely to be heightened.

Wet or deep kissing (frenching) when ulcers and cuts are present on the mouth and/or tongue.

Safer sex

Penetrative sex, assuming a condom is properly used. Specially strengthened condoms are available if required. Condoms and spermicides with non-oxynol 9 are preferred as this spermicide appears to deactivate HIV.

Hugging, caressing, petting.

Kissing, licking, nibbling (the skin is not to be broken).

Mutual masturbation.

Solo masturbation.

Body rubbing ('frotage') and massage.

Sex toys, providing they are not shared.

Erotica (books, videos, magazines, fantasy).

Dirty talking (coprolalia).

Bondage (the skin is not to be broken by whipping/spanking, etc.)

These safer sex activities all assume that the skin of both partners is healthy and unbroken.

Comment

The list is not intended to be definitive and only refers to the most well known sexual activities. If in any doubt consult your local AIDS line or national organisations such as the Terrence Higgins Trust, Scottish AIDS Monitor, Body Positive, or Frontliners.

An inventive enjoyable safer love life and sex life will be very rewarding and will minimise the transmission of HIV considerably.

Appendix C

Safer drug use

Advice on drug abstinence co-existing with an alternative intervention strategy such as advice on drug-taking risk reduction may at first seem quite contradictory. Evidence suggests, however, that drug workers and agencies can play a vital role in minimising the spread of HIV and hepatitis by accepting that, if and when a person becomes unable to stop taking drugs, they should be encouraged to take these drugs as safely as possible in ways that will not lead them to contract HIV and hepatitis or risk spreading these viruses to other people.

Advice

1. Drug abstinence

Drug taking can cause many problems. The healthiest solution is to avoid getting a 'high' by drugs and to try and find other ways and activities to achieve the sought-for excitement and elation. Drugs are on the whole immune-suppressive. Therefore, for those with HIV, there is a greater risk of precipitating ARC and AIDS by continuing to use drugs and alcohol. (Some evidence suggests that the use of drugs can lead to a T4 cell reduction. These cells are not only attacked by the virus but also orchestrate the immune system functioning.) Giving up drugs and staying drug free is not easy. Therefore, the user should be advised not to 'go it alone' but to seek help and counselling from drug agencies and self-help groups.

2. Drug taking

If drugs are to continue to be used then, if at all possible, they should be taken by other methods than injecting. Sniffing, smoking and ingesting drugs (where possible) are all safer methods and contain no risk of HIV infection. It should also be remembered that alongside the risk of contracting HIV and hepatitis by injecting and sharing drug equipment, the process of injecting can carry other risks, notably:

Ulcers and abscesses - caused either by missing the vein altogether when injecting or by using body tissue irritants such as ground-up chalk-based drugs or drug bulkers such as talc, sugar etc. The use of non-sterile injecting equipment and water to dissolve drugs can also lead to abscess formation.

Gangrene (caused by injecting into an artery instead of a vein) and Septicaemia (blood poisoning).

It is also easier to overdose by injecting, especially when the purity and strength of the drug being injected is not known by the user (and in many instances the supplier).

3. Injecting drugs

For those who, nevertheless, have decided to inject their drugs, the following advice can be given:

Always obtain your own needles and injecting equipment (syringes, bowls, spoons etc). NEVER SHARE. A fresh set of needles and syringes should ideally be used every time there is a 'fix' and every attempt should be made to obtain these from chemists, surgical suppliers and needle exchange schemes where they exist locally. These outlets will invariably be able to receive the used 'drug equipment' for disposal so as to avoid the risks of 'equipment' being used by other drug takers. Never dispose of needles and syringes in ways that could cause danger to children in particular and to the community in general.

Where it is not possible to obtain fresh injecting equipment easily it is possible safely to clean the equipment, spoons and bowls.

There has been a major debate over whether injecting equipment can be boiled or cleaned by using bleach and water. Both methods can destroy HIV and hepatitis but the former method is fraught with difficulties as some brands of syringes distort and perish as a result of boiling. The Public Health Laboratory service in Britain is examining this debate at the moment but initial advice given would seem to suggest that needles and syringes can be disinfected by the following procedure:.

(a) Flush out the syringe with cold water.

(b) Draw up undiluted domestic bleach into the syringe, then squirt it out.

(c) Repeat the above process at least twice.

(d) Flush syringe again at least twice with water.

If the syringe is not going to be used again for some while it should be filled with water to prevent any residual blood coagulating.

Bowls and spoons used for mixing drugs prior to injecting should be washed out in hot water and either domestic bleach or washing up liquid.

4. Safer sex

Even if the methods of drug taking are relatively safe, HIV can still be passed on through certain sexual activities (see *Appendix B*). Safer sex guidelines should therefore always be followed alongside safer drug use guidelines.

Key to Network Diagrams

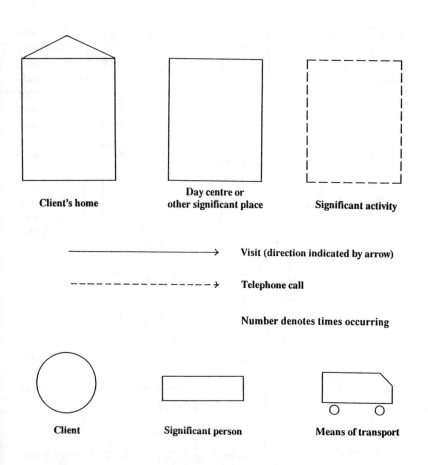

Client's home

Day centre or
other significant place

Significant activity

Visit (direction indicated by arrow)

Telephone call

Number denotes times occurring

Client

Significant person

Means of transport

Appendix E - Sample Diary Form

DH3(P)

DIARY KEPT AT HOME

NAME .... FOR .... DAY DATE ....

List events or activities you can remember while you were at home (or hostel etc.)	Who were you with? If lots of people name important people. (If necessary, explain who they are)
What Happened Today:	
1. DURING THE MORNING	
2. DURING THE AFTERNOON	
3. DURING THE EVENING OR NIGHT	

Did you go out anywhere today? Who with? How did you travel?

PLACES VISITED	WHO WITH?	HOW DID YOU TRAVEL	EVENT OR ACTIVITY	WHO ELSE DID YOU MEET
4. ALL DAY				
OR MORNING				
AFTERNOON				
EVENING OR NIGHT				

5. DID ANYTHING HAPPEN TODAY THAT YOU WANT TO COMMENT ON FURTHER?

Glossary

1. Medical terminology

AIDS - Acquired Immune Deficiency Syndrome

ARC - AIDS Related Complex (or Condition)

AZT - Azidothymidine (Zidovudine or 'Retrovir', trade name)

CMV - Cytomegalovirus

HIV - Human Immuno Deficiency Virus (formerly known as LAV, ARV or HTLV 3)

KS - Kaposi's Sarcoma.

PCP - Pneumocystis Carinii Pneumonia.

PGL - Persistent Generalised Lymphadenopathy.

2. Drug terminology

Amphetamine - stimulant drug illegally found usually in powder form (injected or smoked). Found also in tablet form and abused as pep pill ('speed')

Barbiturates - hypnosedative drugs (taken orally or injected)

Benzodiazepines (minor tranquillisers taken to relieve anxiety or aid sleep - taken orally in tablet or occasionally as a mixture)

Buprenorphine - Temgesic (trade name) - a strong analgesic for the relief of moderate to severe pain (taken orally or by injecting)

Cannabis - relaxing mild intoxicant from the 'Cannabis Sativa' plant found as resin, ('Hash'), dried leaf and stalks ('marihuana', 'grass') or oil. (Cannabis is usually smoked, sometimes taken orally.)

Chlordiazepoxide - trade name 'Librium', a minor tranquiliser (taken orally)

Cocaine - Cocaine Hydrochloride - stimulant drug (sniffed or injected). Note also use of freebase cocaine ('crack') - cocaine blended with baking powder.

Codeine Linctus - diluted mixture of codeine taken orally as cough suppressant. (One of a number of 'over the counter' drugs containing diluted codeine, morphine or opium - note also 'Actifed', 'Gee's Linctus', 'Collis Brown mixture', 'Kaolin and Morphine' mixture.)

Dihydrocodeine 'DF118s' - analgesic (taken orally)

Diazepam - trade name 'Valium', 2, 5, 10 mg., a minor tranquiliser (taken orally).

Dipipanone Hydrochloride - Diconal (trade name) - synthetic opiate analgesic with anti-emetic action (injected).

Heroin - an opiate in powder form produced from morphine and twice as potent (injected, sniffed, smoked and inhaled ('chasing the dragon')).

LSD - Lysergic Acid Diethylamide - highly potent synthetic hallucinogenic drug. A white crystalline material liquified and injected into tablets, paper and taken orally.

Palfium - potent analgesic for relief of severe pain, 5 mg or 10 mg (peach Palfium) - (injected).

Pethidine - synthetic opiate analgesic often given at child birth (taken orally).

Physeptone - Methadone (trade name) - drug mixture usually prescribed for opiate dependence (taken orally).

Temazepam - minor tranquiliser with short half life, 10 or 20 mg. (taken orally or by injecting).

3. Social Terminology.

HIV positive (HIV + ve). On testing, antibodies to HIV shown to be present. Therefore, also known as antibody positive or seropositive.

HIV negative (HIV - ve). No antibodies shown. Also known as antibody negative or seronegative.

Serostatus - the state of being HIV positive or HIV negative.

IDU - Injecting drug user. (*Note* the term IVDA is often used - referring to 'Intravenous Drug Abuser'.) This term should not be used as a composite, excluding as it does intramuscular and subcutaneous (under the skin - 'skin-popping') drug injecting methods.

'Buddies' - supporters and counselling volunteers who often work with AIDS agencies.

'People living with AIDS' - to be preferred to labelling and negative phrases such as AIDS victims, sufferers etc or impersonal abbreviations as PWA (see *Chapter 2*).

4. AIDS organisations.

THT - Terrence Higgins Trust
SAM - Scottish AIDS Monitor
'Frontliners'
'Mainliners'   }   British National HIV-AIDS Agencies
'Body Positive'

5. Drug Organisations.

A.A. - Alcoholics Anonymous.

N.A. - Narcotics Anonymous